"David is an inspiration to our team and is a n[...] fight. He is a physically strong and courageous man, but he will tell you that his spirit to fight this awful disease and make a difference is only by the grace of God. . . . David is truly fighting his Goliath, but as Sir Isaac Newton once said, 'If I have seen further it is by standing on the shoulders of giants.' David is my giant and I can clearly see further because he is in my life and the future looks brighter for us all."

—**Andrew Bishop**, CEO/Executive Producer, Bishop-Lyons Entertainment

"I've known few men as driven as Dave Lyons. Dave's entrepreneurial passion has led to his great success in several companies. With this passion, combined with a strong desire to share the Good News of the Gospel, you have a winning combination of blessing and outreach. . . . Dave's transparency in his personal battle will serve to connect, give hope, and encourage others in the struggles they are facing."

—**Stan Dennis**, National Director, FivestarMan.com

"As a champion professional bodybuilder who has trained for over 40 years, I know the drive, determination, and intensity it takes to train and compete in the sport. It is amazing that David Lyons, diagnosed with multiple sclerosis and over 50 years old, is able to push himself through this exhausting regime that, even for a young, healthy man, would be difficult to undertake."

—**Ed Corney**, former IFBB pro bodybuilder

"I have been Dave's training partner for a while now, training 4-5 days per week together. I have trained with many individuals but Dave definitely stands alone. Despite having MS, he is the most intense training partner I have ever had. Dave and I push to limits I never would have thought possible, and this is training with a guy 20 years older than me who has MS! I don't look at Dave as a man fighting MS. I look at Dave as the best training partner I could have."

—**Frank Duran**, Certified Fitness Trainer

"To see David reach his goal and step on stage at that competition was one of the most rewarding things I have experienced in my fitness career. . . . I have grown as a person as well as a trainer for having been through this challenge with David. I am proud to call David a friend, and truly enjoy watching him continually make strides in his battle against multiple sclerosis."

—**Darren Barnes**, Certified Fitness Trainer and competitive bodybuilder

"David is on a mission and nothing will stop him. God has set him on fire for his work here on this earth and David is running at full steam to accomplish it. This is a modern-day David vs. Goliath story. This time it is David Lyons vs. multiple sclerosis. Instead of a slingshot, his weapon of choice is iron and lots of it. Instead of settling for a wheel chair, he chose the gym. Bold, outspoken, and sometimes outrageous, David Lyons is a bright light in a dark world. Be encouraged by his life, his example, his will power, and his faith. Like David, use life's obstacles as fuel to light you on fire for the work the Lord has for you!"

—**John Rowley**, author of *The Power of Positive Fitness*

"I truly admire David's mission to inspire other people around the world who also have MS to become more physically fit and active. I have committed to help David through every step of the way to realize his dream of becoming a champion bodybuilder once again. I fully support the MS Bodybuilding Challenge and his newly formed MS Fitness Challenge. Together we can make a big difference."

—**Michael Torchia**, former champion bodybuilder, Mr. Teenage New York and Mr. California, founder of Operation Fitness

"David Lyons' amazing life is an unwavering and truly uplifting fight filled with triumph that will enlighten you and hit you profoundly. David teaches us to handle the 'Goliaths' in our own lives."

—**Tomaczek Bednarek**, award-winning producer and singer-songwriter

DAVID'S GOLIATH

WINNING THE BATTLE AGAINST ALL ODDS

DAVID LYONS

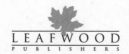

LEAFWOOD
PUBLISHERS

DAVID'S GOLIATH

Winning the Battle against All Odds

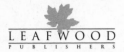

Copyright 2013 by David Lyons

ISBN 978-0-89112-409-2
LCCN 2012043478

Printed in the United States of America

LIBRARY OF CONGRESS CATALOGING-IN-PUBLICATION DATA
Lyons, David, 1958-
  David's goliath : winning the battle against all odds / David Lyons.
     pages cm
  Includes bibliographical references and index.
  ISBN 978-0-89112-409-2 (alk. paper)
  1. Lyons, David, 1958---Health. 2. Multiple sclerosis--Patients--Biography. 3. Bodybuilders--United States--Biography. I. Title.
  RC377.L96 2013
  616.8'340092--dc23
  [B]
                                                            2012043478

Cover design by Thinkpen Design, LLC
Interior text design by Sandy Armstrong

Leafwood Publishers is an imprint of
Abilene Christian University Press
1626 Campus Court
Abilene, Texas 79601

1-877-816-4455
www.leafwoodpublishers.com

13 14 15 16 17 18 / 7 6 5 4 3 2 1

This book is dedicated to my wife, Kendra,
who married me even though she knew that every day of our lives together
would involve a battle against multiple sclerosis. Kendra is more than a
blessing to me and everyone she touches, and I am proud to have her by my
side for life's journey. Kendra, I love you more than words can say.

To my parents, Simon and Shirley,
who have always been there for me over every mountain
I have chosen to climb.

To my children, Deric Brandon, Anna Christine, and Dean Austin.
I love you three, and I am proud of who you are becoming.

To all of the people who have stood by me
and who remain by my side in this journey—
know how much I cherish your teamwork and friendship.

Finally, this book is also dedicated to every MS patient in the world.
You inspire me to keep pushing and to never quit.
My prayers are with you all.

TABLE OF CONTENTS

ACKNOWLEDGMENTS

I would like to thank the following individuals and organizations for their support and contributions:

The Fellowship of Christian Athletes (FCA), who, from the beginning of my journey, gave me the platform to express my love for Christ and allowed me to inspire others—with special thanks to Jimmy Page, who initiated my involvement with their ministry.

The National MS Society, which allowed me to share my story with other MS patients and inspire them to reach for their dreams. Thank you for honoring me with the Milestone Award.

Leafwood Publishers, who had enough faith in my story to publish this book.

John Rowley, who pushed me to share my story with the world and opened the door for me to do so.

Jill Lee, who helped get my words and thoughts into this book with eloquence.

Darren Barnes, who saw my determination to stand on a bodybuilding stage, grabbed hold of that will, and helped the dream become a reality.

The Bishop-Lyons Entertainment team—Andrew and Lane Bishop, John Spagnola, and Kendall Lamkin—who stand by me, encourage me, and allow me the ability to spend as much time in the gym as I need to.

All the sponsors, contributors, and trainers who helped me battle my disease through the MS Bodybuilding Challenge.

My parents, Simon and Shirley Lewenberg, whose love guided and supported me to become the man of strength and willpower I am today.

My children, Deric, Anna, and Dean, who inspire me and fuel me to be the greatest example a father can be to his kids.

My wife, Kendra, who endures this journey with me each and every day. Without her support, love, and dedication, this book would not have been written.

And, most importantly, to Jesus Christ, my Lord and Savior who, without His grace, love, strength, and guidance, I would not have the ability to achieve life's great victories or be a blessing to others.

FOREWORD

Every great competitor loves to be told, "It can't be done." Because at the heart of every athlete is a desire to do the impossible, to overcome the longest odds, to face the greatest opponent—and win. Those four little words—it can't be done—provide all the fuel necessary to stoke the fire within. That's why we love the upset. We love the underdog. And we love the game-winning drive, the buzzer-beater, and the walk-off home run.

In 2006, my friend David Lyons was diagnosed with multiple sclerosis (MS). MS is a disease that affects the brain and spinal cord resulting in loss of muscle control, vision, balance, and sensation (such as numbness). With MS, the nerves of the brain and spinal cord are damaged by one's own immune system when it mistakenly attacks normal tissues.

He was told by doctors that he would quickly deteriorate, need a walker, and eventually end up in a wheelchair. In 2008, he decided to fight back. He responded by setting the impossible goal of competing in a bodybuilding competition at the age of fifty. Everyone said, you guessed it, "It can't be done." His doctors told him he was crazy and that intense physical training would be detrimental to his condition. But, to everyone's amazement, David competed and received a standing ovation to go along with his Most Inspirational Bodybuilder trophy.

If that were the end of the story, it would be a good story, but not a great story. A good story only becomes inspirational when it's about something bigger. David wanted his trial to produce a testimony about the greatness and goodness of his God. He knew that this test had the potential to transform him and encourage others. He began to trust not only that everything happens for a reason but that everything happens "for us to reason." There was truth to be discovered. He chose to believe that there was purpose in his pain.

> Consider it pure joy, my brothers and sisters, whenever you face trials of many kinds, because you know that the testing of your faith produces perseverance. Let perseverance finish its work so that you may be mature and complete, not lacking anything. (James 1:2–4)

In order for God to truly transform us, it takes time, pressure, and heat. That's how uncommonly brilliant diamonds are formed out of the common element, carbon. God uses trials to make us unshakeable and Him unmistakable. Under pressure, our faith is forced into the open and shows its true colors.

My friend David discovered a renewed sense of urgency to pursue Christ and make him known. He reconnected with the Fellowship of Christian Athletes (FCA) and began telling his story at local high schools, colleges, camps, and events. He became a passionate and inspirational writer, writing several FCA Daily Impact Plays that are read by thousands. His writing has also been featured in the FCA Athlete's Bible.

He has inspired thousands to seize the day, trust in God, and live for His glory. He has a passion for using the platform of sports to lead others to a relationship with Jesus. The more "heat and pressure" he felt, the more "heart and presence" of God he relied on. He let the power of God push him to train and comfort him in his pain.

It is likely that each one of us will face our own tests and trials. No one is exempt from hardship. How we respond to that kind of adversity reveals our character. Character is uncovered in crisis and formed in the fire. It is both revealed and refined. When we are squeezed, what comes out reveals what's inside.

I know David as a great man of God and an overcomer. His story will inspire you to be the man or woman God has designed you to be. And when you face adversity so big it scares you, and everyone tells you "It can't be done," just smile and remember this one thing—nothing is impossible with God.

Win Today,
Jimmy Page

Fellowship of Christian Athletes (FCA), VP of Field Ministry, Executive Director Health & Fitness; coauthor of two best-selling books, *WisdomWalks* and *WisdomWalks Sports*

www.fca.org
www.wisdomwalks.org

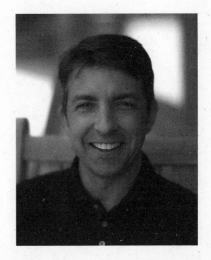

From Wikipedia, the free encyclopedia

Multiple sclerosis (abbreviated MS, known as disseminated sclerosis or encephalomyelitis disseminata) is an inflammatory disease in which the fatty myelin sheaths around the axons of the brain and spinal cord are damaged, leading to demyelination and scarring as well as a broad spectrum of signs and symptoms. Disease onset usually occurs in young adults, and it is more common in women. It has a prevalence that ranges between 2 and 150 per 100,000. MS was first described in 1868 by Jean-Martin Charcot.

MS affects the ability of nerve cells in the brain and spinal cord to communicate with each other effectively. Nerve cells communicate by sending electrical signals called action potentials down long fibers called axons, which are contained within an insulating substance called myelin. In MS, the body's own immune system attacks and damages the myelin. When myelin is lost, the axons can no longer effectively conduct signals. The name multiple sclerosis refers to scars (scleroses—better known as plaques or lesions) particularly in the white matter of the brain and spinal cord, which is mainly composed of myelin. Although much is known about the mechanisms involved in the disease process, the cause remains unknown. Theories include genetics or infections. Different environmental risk factors have also been found.

Almost any neurological symptom can appear with the disease, and often progresses to physical and cognitive disability. MS takes several forms, with new symptoms occurring either in discrete attacks (relapsing forms) or slowly accumulating over time (progressive forms). Between attacks, symptoms may go away completely, but permanent neurological problems often occur, especially as the disease advances.

There is no known cure for multiple sclerosis. Treatments attempt to return function after an attack, prevent new attacks, and prevent disability. MS medications can have adverse effects or be poorly tolerated, and many patients pursue alternative treatments, despite the lack of supporting scientific study. The prognosis is difficult to predict; it depends on the subtype of the disease, the individual patient's disease characteristics, the initial symptoms and the degree of disability the person experiences as time advances. Life expectancy of people with MS is 5 to 10 years lower than that of the unaffected population. (http://en.wikipedia.org/wiki/Multiple_sclerosis)

Chapter 1

THE ATTACK

Some days I wake up and wonder whose life this is. Years ago, if someone would have asked me what I thought I would be doing in my fifties, this would not have been it. Who would ever have thought that a man diagnosed with multiple sclerosis would be training to compete in his second bodybuilding contest at the age of fifty-three? If you heard that, you'd probably think he was crazy. I know I would. And I certainly would never have guessed that the man would be me.

As I struggle with things that healthy people take for granted, I fix my mind on the goal and push past the pain, numbness, tingling, lack of coordination, and other "fun" symptoms of MS. I strain to get out of bed, shower, take my supplements, and hit the gym, and I wonder why I'm compelled to take this on. Why has the Lord chosen this road for me? That's not an easy question, and it doesn't have an easy answer. But

I believe this journey is guided by the Lord and ordained by Him. It's a voyage not unlike those of other athletes intent on breaking records or inventors who work to create amazing inventions. My undertaking is an odds-defying trial focused on defeating a disease that I was told would defeat me. As I think of the diagnoses and prognosis handed to me by experts, I ponder the events, trials, and milestones I have encountered along the way. This is a story of challenge, of battle, and of the road to victory.

On August 22, 2009, I stood on a bodybuilding stage doing what naysayers said I couldn't, and I did so despite the great fear of being humiliated by the competition. As the crowd cheered and the lights blinded my view, I had no idea what was going on around me, but I knew it had to be good. When I finished my final posing routine, I knew I'd accomplished something big. Later, I was told by my wife, Kendra, that I had received a standing ovation from the packed auditorium.

I felt in my heart that the Lord had brought me to that day for a purpose. After all, it had only been a few years earlier, in June of 2006, when my life had been forever changed and I had been dealt a new set of cards that made me the Rocky Balboa of my own life. For the first time, I became the underdog instead of the highly favored contender. My past successes were no good to me anymore. I was no longer the David Lyons who could conquer the world. . . . Or was I?

---   ▧   ▧   ▧   ---

The prelude to the worst episode of my life began in March 2006. I woke up one beautiful Orlando, Florida, morning feeling great. I mean, what could be wrong when I was living the dream in the Disney-built community of Celebration? That morning, with nothing on my mind except getting my workout done, I headed to the gym just like I'd done six days a week for many years.

About thirty minutes into my triceps workout, something happened, and I can only describe it as a sharp, burning pain in my left shoulder. But like many of us hard-headed competitors do, I kept going in the workout, ignoring the feeling even as it traveled down my left arm and into my fingers.

I moved on to my biceps workout thinking the pain was stemming from some kind of pinched nerve in my neck or shoulder. For a brief moment I even considered that I might be having a heart attack, but I quickly dismissed that idea since there was no tightness in my chest. Plus, I was David Lyons; I didn't have heart attacks.

The painful burning sensation remained in my left shoulder and arm even after the workout ended. It stayed with me for a week or so, and, as a Christian man, I prayed to the Lord and asked Him to alleviate the issue. Instead of going away, however, the pain began to spread to my lower back, and I also developed new symptoms of tingling and numbness. At this point, I was convinced that it was some sort of sciatic nerve problem that was the result of overtraining, and I refused to see a doctor, believing that God would heal me shortly. Why wouldn't He? That had always been the case before. I rarely ever got sick, and, when I did, it only lasted for a day or so before it was over and I was back to normal.

As the days turned into weeks, though, I began to experience numbness all over my body. I couldn't even feel myself urinating. My legs were no longer cooperating, and I was struggling to walk. Every night I woke up in a panic wondering what was really happening to me. I couldn't wrap my head around the idea that it was anything more than a temporary condition and that it would eventually subside. I prayed for it to end and to wake up normal again in the morning.

The severity of my condition really hit me hard one day when I went swimming with my three children, Deric, Anna, and Dean. I tried to get out of the pool but was unable to raise my legs onto the outside edge. Dean, my youngest, literally had to pull me out. When I tried to stand, I ended up slamming my knees on the concrete deck because I had no feeling in my lower extremities. The strange thing was that I couldn't feel the pain of the impact even though both knees were bleeding. I knew then this was more than a simple nerve condition.

The timing for the situation was terrible. In 2002, just a few years earlier, I had decided to begin a new career as the creator and producer of television and film projects, which was an unknown field to me. As with all of my endeavors to date, it couldn't be done. Without connections or experience, I would never make it in the entertainment business, especially living in Florida. But that was just what I'd needed to hear in order to take it on.

Through much work, a lot of learning, and tons of mistakes, I finally got two TV projects and an animated film moving forward. I'd made a deal with Octagon, a leading sports entertainment marketing company, and with FOX Sports on two sports reality competition shows I'd created; the official paperwork to produce and air the shows was in process. I was also scheduled to head out to Hollywood for five days to pitch my animated children's project, *Creepers*, to TV networks and distribution companies. But here I was, stressed and straining to even move my legs.

The trip to California had been planned for more than a month and included meetings that had taken weeks to get scheduled. Plus, one of my mentors, Mark Simon, had taken time out from his hectic calendar and was booked to travel with me. I had a choice: cancel this once-in-a-lifetime trip and go to a doctor, or bear with it and get on the plane. I chose to get on the plane.

When I arrived at the Orlando airport on April 16, I was barely able to coordinate my steps. I could hardly hold my briefcase or pull my suitcase, and Mark had to help me board the plane. It was a five-hour direct flight, so I talked to Mark and prepared for the meetings to keep my mind off what was happening to my body.

As we approached Los Angeles International Airport, I could see the concern on Mark's face. I knew he was thinking, "Is Dave nuts? How is he going to go through these meetings when he can't even get on and off a plane?" As we landed, he looked at me and, just as I thought he would, asked, "Dave, how are you going to do this? Can you make it through this week?"

I looked Mark in the eyes and replied, "We've come this far and have both done so much. I have no choice but to do this."

The plane landed at LAX, and we were off to the races. I, however, wasn't running anywhere. Mark helped me off the plane, down to baggage claim, in and out of the rental car, and into our hotel. Simple things were monumental obstacles for me. Mark managed to get me to our room, but I was exhausted from my body's battle to keep moving. After settling in and prepping for our meetings, we made it an early evening to bed.

I awoke the next morning feeling even worse than I had the night before. The combination of stress from travel, not knowing what was happening to me physically, and the upcoming barrage from network executives had taken a tremendous toll on me. Uncoordinated and in pain, I held onto walls and maneuvered my way into the shower and then dressed for the long day ahead, all the while praying for the strength to remain mobile for the next five days.

In our first meeting we found success. *Creepers*, which got its title from the main characters of lizards and bugs, was a hit with one distributor, and she made an offer to green-light the project. That great news gave me the boost I needed to keep going and keep pitching. We still had a long week ahead, and we needed to keep our remaining meetings in case this deal fell through.

The five days were grueling. Getting in and out of the rental car, going up and down elevators, and navigating stairs were all but impossible. Mark became my assistant, both helping me walk and carrying my briefcase. As the meetings went by, I could see that his concern was growing and that he wasn't convinced that my condition was a simple ailment or injury.

As I replay the trip in my mind, I see it as a short film—a montage of pain, numbness, and apprehension. My faith helped me get through the fear, but it was difficult to stay positive. I knew that I was ignoring something I shouldn't have been ignoring; yet, three thousand miles from home, I felt I had no choice but to keep going.

In an effort to keep up with my normal life and prove that I was okay, I even attempted to work out one morning in the hotel gym. That was a disaster. Because I couldn't feel myself using the equipment, Mark had to help me out of one of the machines and back to the room.

I felt bad about putting Mark through all of that uncertainty. Inside, I questioned whether he had made the right decision to come with me and wondered whether I was going to collapse or die on him. While we've talked about it some since then, I can still only imagine what was going through the poor guy's mind as he watched me struggle and strain. Still, we both made the decision to forge ahead in the trip and agreed to do what we could.

The evening before our last pitch day, Mark had a social event to attend, and, because of my condition, I passed. Instead, I stayed in the hotel room and watched Carrie Underwood win *American Idol* while slowly slipping further into an abyss of physical deterioration. By the time Mark came back, I was having trouble breathing and couldn't even feel my chest moving up and down. I was virtually immobilized in the bed trying to force the breath in and out of my lungs. My chest moved up in a labored manner and dropped rapidly down as the air left. All I could do was lie there asking the Lord to get me through the night and to do the breathing for me while I slept.

I turned to Mark, who was sitting on his bed, and told him I might not make it through the night. He wondered if he should call 911 or take me to a local hospital, but I told him to let whatever happened happen and that we'd figure it out in the morning. I had faith in Christ and believed I would be going to a better place if I died anyway. I was honestly more afraid of being crippled than I was of dying.

For reasons only He knows, God kept me alive, and I made it through the night. In fact, that morning, I actually felt better and in greater control of my breathing. It was our last day of meetings, and we would be going home that day.

Once we were ready, Mark and I headed out to meet with the creator and producer of the animated hit show *Rugrats* at his home in Malibu Lake. When we pulled up to his beautiful waterfront mansion, I saw something that made me think twice about getting out of the car. The home was set atop a small hill with more than thirty steep steps leading up to the front door. Mark and I looked at each other both thinking, *I can't believe this.* I just told him to grab my arm and steady me up the path.

I managed to drag my legs up each agonizing step to the front door, but I felt like a drunk trying to walk the line during a sobriety test. It reminded me of when I had watched the Jerry Lewis telethons for muscular dystrophy (MD) and observed the patients' uncoordinated movements. That was me. As I struggled up the stairs, I wondered if I actually had MD, but of course I didn't say anything.

After we'd finally made it up the last step and into the spacious house, we found out that the producer was stuck in another meeting across town and would have to leave us with his assistant. I was disappointed and annoyed. We left our pitch presentation with her, turned to leave, and headed back down all those steps. One more day was gone, and we only had LAX to tackle.

Getting around LAX and onto the plane was demanding, but the five-hour flight back to Orlando was downright arduous. As I sat in my seat, I began to experience the worst pain I'd felt yet. It was an exaggerated sensation like what you get when you fall asleep on your arm and wake up with the feeling of pins and needles. I couldn't feel any movement, but I could certainly feel intense pain. The awful tingling stemmed from my chest and down to my feet and didn't let up for the entire trip. I kept trying to move my toes to make sure I wouldn't become completely paralyzed. The only way I knew they were responding was to see my shoes move.

The flight couldn't end fast enough. I felt like I was being tortured to some extent, and I was scared. Any excitement I felt about the production deal was overshadowed by the inner dread of going home to face my medical fate. My worry increased with each minute, and I started to believe I had made a mistake by risking my life for this business trip. I wanted to say I was excited to walk away from the journey with a distribution deal for *Creepers*, but I wasn't really walking. It was so bittersweet. I had the offer I wanted, but I was numb from the chest down and struggling to maneuver into the taxi for a ride home.

Even though I knew better, I refused to see a doctor when I got home. I took matters into my own hands, again, not wanting to believe this was happening to me. I was acting like a child who closes his eyes and believes no one can see him. Now at home, I was in a state of artificial safety. You'd think a person with numbness from his chest down who could barely coordinate his legs would immediately go to a doctor, but I just continued to believe that the Lord would heal me miraculously and that I would wake up one morning with nothing wrong. Through this experience, I came to understand that there is a difference between faith and stupidity. Clearly, I was in denial.

I tried everything in my power to relieve the numbness and other symptoms. I even went out and bought a thousand-dollar massage chair hoping it would generate some sort of feeling, but it actually created more pain. I sat in hot whirlpool spas, iced my spine, and took every supplement known to man if it claimed to help nerve damage. Nothing.

Finally, after a month of following my own self-help plan and spending hours asking God to just take it away, I realized that my condition was actually getting worse by the day. It was now late May, and I knew I needed to get to a doctor—and soon.

Because my doctor was a general practitioner and didn't specialize in neurological disorders, he wasn't sure what was happening to me other than that it wasn't just a pinched nerve or sciatic issue. While I was there, he did the strangest test on me. After warning me that it would be an awkward test, he hit the top of my head with his palm—quite forcefully—and asked what I felt. My response was that it hurt my head! I thought to myself, *He has no clue what he's doing.* Looking back, I laugh at my prideful, angry reaction. Because I was so mad that he'd done such a ridiculous test, I never even thought to ask what the heck he was trying to find out.

Apparently he had been looking for a cause. During the office exam, he asked me if I had ever been in an accident that had involved a head injury or if I'd ever experienced trauma in that area. When I disclosed my past as a fighter, both in and out of the ring, his eyes widened. He thought that maybe all of the punishment I had taken over the years had finally caught up with me. He concluded that what was happening was likely related to nerve damage that had accumulated as my brain had repeatedly struck the inside of my skull every time I was hit. It made sense to me.

With his assumptions regarding my condition, he ordered an MRI of my brain to see whether the damage was related to my years as an amateur boxer. This was the first mistake in the process—aside from my dragging my feet in going to the doctor. What we would later find out was that my entire spine should have been examined in order to accurately test his theory. Instead, we proceeded to focus on the brain.

Because I have a great deal of claustrophobia when it comes to enclosed spaces, the tight, confining MRI machine wasn't an option for me; so, I went for an open MRI instead. Once the test was done, all I could do was wait.

On June 6, 2006, our phone rang and Helen, my wife at the time, answered. It was my doctor calling with the MRI results and telling Helen that she needed to rush me to the Florida Hospital Cancer Institute in Orlando, where I was already preregistered. The doctor said that the MRI showed a mass in my brain that was likely a brain tumor and possibly cancer. It was imperative that I be admitted and have a cancer specialist diagnose the results of the MRI. The doctor was concerned that I might have waited too long and that my life was now in jeopardy.

My whole family was shocked. My sister-in-law, who lived across the street, frantically raced over to watch my children so that my wife could drive me to the hospital. Nobody really knew what was happening; we all just knew I needed to get to the hospital quickly.

While everyone else's panic buttons had been pushed, I, for some reason, was surprisingly calm and resigned in the situation. My own health didn't concern me much, and, since my marriage wasn't in a good place, my main concern was about my children and how their lives would be affected without a father. No, I didn't want to die, but I was secure in my faith and in God's plan for me—be it here on earth or with Him in heaven.

Once we got to the hospital, I sat for several hours in their admitting area just praying and thinking, until I was finally brought up into a private room on the cancer unit floor. By now it was late in the evening, and no testing could be performed until the morning. They did start an IV full of a very strong, prednisone-based drug to help with the inflammation of the nervous system and relieve some of the numbness and paralysis. The nurse also explained that she would have to insert a catheter so I could urinate since I was having difficulty walking and couldn't feel my extremities. Not being interested in that idea, I told her I would get myself to the bathroom, numbness or not. She then gave me the alternative, handing me a urine container that I would have to fill every day in order to eliminate enough to keep my body from being poisoned. It was the container or the catheter—period. I chose the container.

I used every bit of mental strength I had and asked the Lord for the power to get to the bathroom to do what needed to be done. He always gave me the ability. With no feeling in my lower body, I managed to walk, holding onto anything I could and dragging an IV pole behind me. Every day I stumbled my way to the bathroom and steadied myself to urinate, shower, and do the normal bathroom tasks. I wasn't willing to be catheterized, and I refused to be cared for as an invalid. I kept telling myself I was strong and healthy—that I could do this without extra care. To me, the strength I was using was a gift from God, and when God wants to make a point, He makes it. He was exclaiming His will!

That evening, though, as I lay in the hospital bed, I finally realized where I was and what was happening. I had to face the fact that this could seriously be the end of my life, or at least the end of my life as I had known it. My mind was jumping all over the place. I kept thinking, *What's going to happen next? How will I get past this? What is God doing?* I wrestled between faith and bursts of panic. Mostly, I believed that something would change the situation for the better. I just believed that I had so much more to accomplish in life. My career in entertainment was starting to develop, and I just couldn't see how God would want to take me now, when we had worked so hard to get to that point. Confused and distressed, I took my sleeping pill and drifted off.

Morning came, and the oncologist came in to discuss the MRI results and my options. With a stoic expression, he began to tell my wife and me that what he saw on the MRI was a brain tumor that looked cancerous. He would not know for sure until he operated, though, and I needed to get into surgery immediately. Cancer or not, the mass had to be removed.

My first reaction was that I wasn't going to let anyone cut into my brain to remove anything. I asked him the odds of removing the mass successfully with no complications, and his response was alarming. He said that because the tumor was in a volatile place near nerves, it would leave me semiparalyzed even if he removed it with no complications. He also said the operation was risky and that I had a fifty percent chance of survival. Without the surgery, though, I wouldn't live much longer anyway.

"Let me get this straight, doc," I said. "You're telling me that, no matter what, you have to operate. And if you do, I have a fifty percent chance of dying and a one hundred percent chance of being paralyzed?"

"Yes, that's correct," he replied.

I said, "Then I choose to die. No one is cutting into my brain."

He tried to convince me otherwise, and with a Christian-like manner I told him to back off and get out of my room. My main nurse heard all of this and suggested they call in a neurologist. Fortunately, they had one of the country's top neurological doctors working at their hospital: Dr. Nicholas G. Avgeropoulos, or, as the nurses called him, "Dr. Nic."

With my next exam the following day, I had to get through another night of uncertainty and anxiety. Sleeping pills came in handy, but with the nurses taking vital signs and checking my IV every few hours, sleep gave me no escape. Any peaceful retreat was short-lived, as I would be woken up frequently to face the reality of my nightmare.

The next day, I decided it was time to call everyone I worked with on my entertainment projects and inform them of what was happening. To this point, only family members were aware of my condition and location.

I called my partners from *Creepers* and my FOX shows and let them know I might not be coming out of the hospital the same as I was before—if alive at all. At that moment, I wouldn't be able to think about business, TV shows, films, or anything else except my health. They would just have to move forward without me or let things stand still.

Those were some of the hardest calls I'd ever had to make. Years of hard work in the cutthroat Hollywood machine were about to pay off, and I was just a finger tip's distance away. But I just couldn't worry about it. My focus had to be on my life, my children, and what was going to take place in the hours, days, and weeks ahead. Unsure of how long I had left to live, I couldn't think about months or years. In my heart, though, I believed I was finished whether I lived or not.

Later that day, Dr. Nic came to see me and ordered multiple enclosed MRIs, which were more accurate than open MRIs. He was actually taken aback when he discovered that the oncologist had relied on the findings of an open MRI to make the decision to perform such a risky operation. Dr. Nic was a great man with a terrific demeanor and an entertaining sense of humor. He was positive and upbeat, and he constantly assured me that he would do whatever he could to help me and not suggest any impulsive operations.

I soon was informed that I would need extensive MRI testing on my brain and spine, which would take almost six hours. Because of my claustrophobia, that wasn't going to happen without some sedation. As I was wheeled into the elevator and down hallways to the MRI, my anxiety intensified. When I entered the exam room, the nurse prepped me for an IV of liquid Valium. Once I was injected, I was sent into the MRI tube, which I referred to as a coffin.

I remember the experience, but it seems more like a dream than a reality because of my level of sedation. I wondered when I would be put to sleep, but I never actually was. I was just highly tranquilized and felt like I was in heaven. I do remember them taking me out of the machine to inject die into my veins for specific testing, and I also recall that the Valium began to wear off twice, which made me realize my setting.

When that happened, they had to take me out again and administer more Valium, just as I would start to get upset. Now, I know I'm not the easiest guy to deal with even when I'm comfortable, but six hours in an MRI would rattle anyone's cage.

▩   ▩   ▩

It was late afternoon when the results came in. According to these more accurate MRIs, I had multiple brain and spinal cord lesions—two near my neck and three in various spots on my brain. Lesions are bare spots on the nerves that resemble scars and create a disconnect between the nerves wherever they are located. I had these disconnections disrupting my system in several areas. Apparently, my body was attacking itself in what seemed to be some form of autoimmune response.

Dr. Nic had an idea about what was causing the issue, but he wanted to order more tests, including blood work and a spinal tap, to confirm what he believed. He didn't want to make the same mistake the oncologist had made and deliver a premature diagnosis. After enduring so much improper care, I found it difficult to trust him, but I chose to go with it and to find my peace in the Lord. With faith being all I had to hold on to, I waited for more tests.

It was now day three of my hospital stay, and all I could think about was going home. Instead, I was scheduled for a spinal tap, also called a lumbar puncture (LP). Without getting too technical, an LP is a procedure that is performed when a doctor needs to look at the spinal fluid in order to check for infections, bleeding in the brain, disorders of the central nervous system, or cancers of the brain or spinal cord. A needle is inserted between two lumbar vertebrae to remove a sample of the cerebrospinal fluid that surrounds the brain and spinal cord and protects them from injury. This was certainly not a pleasant experience, but it was necessary in order to get an accurate diagnosis.

Dr. Nic sat me up in my hospital bed with my legs hanging over the side, and had me lean forward onto the back of a chair. He numbed the area and waited for the Lidocaine to set in. I wasn't sure whether I even needed the anesthetic since I was numb everywhere anyway, but it was procedure. He then told me not to move or else he might hit something he shouldn't. That certainly wasn't very reassuring, but he had a great sense of humor and kept me entertained throughout the process.

I tried to relax as much as possible while Dr. Nic carefully put a needle into a space between the bones in my lower back. I felt some pushing, but because of my numbness there was no discomfort. Once it was over, he took his large syringe full of my spinal fluid, told me he would have the results the next day, and left. I faced enduring another day and night without knowing my condition.

On the fourth day, Dr. Nic came to give me the test results and his diagnosis. As usual, he was cheerful and delivered the news in a positive manner, but the news was not positive at all. He informed me that, from what he saw, I had all of the symptoms and signs of multiple sclerosis (MS)—an inflammatory disease in which the myelin sheaths around the axons of the brain and spinal cord are damaged, affecting the ability of nerve cells in the brain and spinal cord to communicate with each other effectively. He did say that it could potentially be a virus since I had never had an attack like this before, but in his opinion, we should discuss the high probability that it was MS.

At the time, I was completely unfamiliar with MS, so I had no idea what it meant except that if what I was going through was due to this disease, I didn't want to have it.

Since I'd claimed to never have had an attack like this before, Dr. Nic wanted to know if I'd experienced any symptoms that might have indicated my development of MS earlier than now. In his years of practice, he had never had a patient be diagnosed with MS so late in life. He also stated that it was rare for a man to experience his first MS attack in his mid-forties. I was forty-seven. MS usually hits people in their early twenties and thirties, but forties is extremely rare. He didn't believe this was a new occurrence in my body and explained that most of the lesions he'd seen in the MRI looked ten to fifteen years old.

I was stunned. How could that be possible? I'd never had an attack of any kind—or had I? I wondered for a moment and tried to recall my past. In order to discuss the subject more thoroughly, Dr. Nic scheduled a time to come back the next day and chat about my history.

I tried to let all of the news set in, but I found it exceedingly difficult to do. I couldn't have multiple sclerosis. No one I knew had it, and I really didn't know anything about it or what it would mean for my life. Confined to my hospital room, I wobbled around, pulling my IV pole and holding onto everything I could to steady myself. I kept telling myself it was just a virus that would go away and never come back. All of the symptoms my body was going through would eventually disappear without a trace, and I would be back in the gym lifting weights again before I knew it. I could not and would not accept the possibility of having MS.

Recalling the event, I can still feel the powerful emotional shock and the obstinate denial in my heart that made me tense with anger. *There must have been a mistake,* I thought. *I can't have MS. I'm too old for that. MS hits people in their twenties and thirties, and I'm just too healthy.*

Once again, night came, and so did the sleeping pills. I escaped to sleep and was relieved from my thoughts.

On the fifth day, I was finally moving more fluidly and feeling better. I was still numb and uncoordinated, but the pain had lessened. Through God's divine power, I had walked without any feeling in my legs and grasped for things without any sensation in my hands. The left side of my body, which had been affected first, was in worse shape than the right side. It had more numbness and pain and experienced more of the pins-and-needles sensation.

While it was still difficult and painful, I was able to move around that day without the same degree of discomfort. I still had an IV pumping me full of medication to keep me stable, which annoyed me. Even though I feared what would happen when it was pulled out, I still counted the minutes until it was gone. Having a needle stuck in my vein and being attached to a pole made me feel bound up, and it intensified my claustrophobia. Knowing I couldn't remove it if I wanted to made me feel caged, and, even if it was helping, I wanted to be free of it.

Dr. Nic walked into the room that day and sat next to me on the bed. I appreciated his disarming jokes about my being his favorite person to see, and that helped prepare me for the history interview. To start, Dr. Nic asked me many questions about my past and urged me to check my memory for clues. He asked about previous head trauma and other possible causes of damage to my brain. He wanted to know if I'd ever lost vision in an eye, slurred my speech, or if I'd lost my balance regularly. My mind swam through my past. *Think, David, think,* I told myself. And then it hit me. It wasn't just one incident; there were many that fit right into his theory.

The first instance that came to mind was from a year before this attack. I had been walking my dog when the vision in my left eye suddenly went black. It was a strange darkness that didn't block all of my sight, just part of it—like there was a black hole whenever I looked to the left. After about fifteen minutes, it was gone.

This weird episode happened a few more times, with each instance happening in close proximity to the others, and then it never happened again. So, as I'd done with most medical issues, I'd ignored it. I have a hard time coming to terms with my own mortality, and I usually choose to discount anything abnormal that happens in my health.

After recalling the vision loss, I thought back even further in my life to times when I'd experienced strange symptoms. I'd lost my balance or stumbled for no apparent reason. People would tell me I was slurring my speech. I would lose my train of thought midstream and grasp for simple words that were typically easy to verbalize. In fact, just before the attack, I had been experienced double-vision while watching TV in bed. I'd always dismissed these occurrences and chalked them up to being punched one too many times in the boxing ring. From what I understood, all fighters had these issues later in life, so why should I be any different?

With the revelation of these new details, a new light was cast on my condition. It was clear that I had indeed experienced episodes of multiple sclerosis–like attacks, and Dr. Nic's suspicions were being confirmed. He explained that because of my consistent exercising over the years and my otherwise great health, my body had been able to fight off major MS attacks for possibly ten to fifteen years, despite the formation of the lesions. Although MS was attacking the myelin sheath of my nerves and causing them to malfunction, I was still able to operate normally and avoid the onslaught of the disease.

Dr. Nic did his best to prepare me for what was ahead in my life as an MS patient, and it didn't sound like a trip to Disney World. It was a progressive disease with no cure, and the best they could do with medication was to try to slow the process down and limit my attacks. With my lack of feeling and other remaining symptoms, Dr. Nic informed me that a walker was a must and that a wheelchair was inevitable.

That was not what I wanted to hear. While trying to digest the information, I still knew one thing. I looked right at him and said, "You don't know my Lord, Jesus Christ, do you?" By His might and power, I said I would overcome this trial and never use a walker or a wheelchair.

I know Dr. Nic thought I was quite unrealistic and still in a state of denial, but he was not about to discourage me from my hard stance of faith. I did, however, see him shake his head as he left.

So, with a diagnosis in place, there was nothing more to do at the hospital. After spending five days at what I jokingly called "Hotel California," I was set to be released the next day. On day six, the nurse entered my room, removed the IV, and had me sign the release papers. While I was elated to be going home, I was still frightened about my future. I prayed for strength and courage as I awaited my chariot to the exit door: a wheelchair. I tried to resist sitting in the wheelchair, but because of hospital policy, which requires all patients to be wheeled out, I didn't have much choice. I fought it for a while until the nurse told me I wouldn't be leaving if I didn't cooperate. Reluctantly, I sat down and let the aide wheel me down the corridor, into the elevator, and through the lobby. But before he could get to front door, I pushed my body up and out of the chair and wobbled my way out through the automatic doors. There was no way I was going out into the world in a wheelchair, and that was final.

Chapter 2

HITTING ROCK BOTTOM

I arrived home from the five-day hospital "vacation" to face my parents, who had been taking care of our children. They all had a thousand questions, and it was exhausting having to relive what had happened and explain the situation. I only wanted to say it once, so I sat everyone down and explained the whats, whys, and hows of the whole ordeal, from the diagnosis to the long-term outlook. My parents cried. They didn't want their seemingly healthy son to have MS. I doubt many parents could have endured the news with dry eyes. My father, a Holocaust survivor, then in his early eighties, and my mother, who was quickly approaching her eighties as well, listened with heavy hearts as I expanded what this all meant.

Knowing that it wasn't easy news for my children to hear, I remained as strong as I could so that they could do the same. They were still quite young at the time. Deric was twelve, Anna was ten, and Dean was seven. They couldn't comprehend the idea of their dad having a disease or even being sick.

In the back of my mind I was still holding onto the possibility that it was a virus, so I put on a false display of optimism. I told them that until I had another attack or unless the symptoms didn't go away, I would continue to believe that I didn't have MS. Not being able to digest anything else, my children agreed with that notion, and my parents reluctantly supported my optimistic façade. Finally, when the briefing was over, I spastically made my way up the stairs to my bedroom to rest. I had much to ponder and very little tolerance to speak to anyone about it anymore. I was drained.

That first night in my bed was brutal. Away from the help of the doctors and nurses, I had no one to lean on for answers and no IV of anti-inflammatory medicine. Sadly, my wife and I had lost all intimacy by that point, and she was unwilling to help. I was alone.

In the deteriorated state of our marriage, my wife, although physically present, had been unsupportive during my hospital stay, and she continued to remain out of touch in what would now be my recovery from the attack. With no feeling in my legs and only a faint ability to hold the steering wheel, I'd even had to drive myself home from the hospital. In my heart, I could sense that the relationship was eventually going to end, but now was not the time. Instead of battling with my wife, I chose to take care of myself and my children as I had always done. The only difference now was that it was going to be far more difficult.

I tried to sleep that first night back, but it wasn't happening. I would nod off into peace only to wake up startled and anxious. During the moments I was asleep, I couldn't feel anything wrong with my body; but the minute I woke up, it hit me that I was numb, in pain, and not the same man I once was. I kept asking God why. I kept praying for answers and for healing. I needed something to hold onto. The thirty-minute bursts of sleep did nothing to relieve my anxiety. The only thing that helped was knowing that God was listening—that He was there and that He had answers. I just wasn't hearing anything yet.

During my first few days of being back home, I sat and read my Bible. I prayed for more answers and watched the time slowly drift away from me. Because I had done well in business, there was money in the bank, but I knew it would eventually dwindle since I couldn't concentrate on anything but what my body was going through.

MS affects a person's cognitive thinking ability, and I was no exception. I easily lost my thoughts and had a difficult time focusing beyond midafternoon when my body would tire from its battle.

A few days later I had a follow-up visit with Dr. Nic. Going in, I was nervous about what he would tell me, assuming the worst and trying to guess what was ahead. As we sat down, we discussed at length what he had discovered in my tests. Every time he mentioned the term multiple sclerosis, though, I would insist that it could still be a virus. Because Dr. Nic was a great doctor and a compassionate man, he didn't want me to have false hope. He tried to take my mind out of the clouds and ground me in what he felt was a certain future. He made it very clear that he believed I had MS, and he shared frankly how the disease would inevitably progress.

Considering the severity of the attack, he did not see the possibility of my symptoms reversing. In his years of experience, he had consistently seen MS patients succumb to using walkers and wheelchairs, especially when they refused to use MS medications. Because there is no cure for MS, medication would be recommended in order to prevent or limit subsequent attacks and slow the progression. I didn't want to hear a word of what I was being told, and I left the appointment angry and frustrated.

            ✦   ✦   ✦

After our appointment, Dr. Nic referred me to a neurologist who specialized in MS. While I liked Dr. Nic a great deal, he practiced out of a location that was too far from my home, which would have limited my ability to see him on a regular basis. The new doctor was located in Celebration Hospital, which was in my neighborhood and only minutes away from my front door. It was a well-run facility, and I made an appointment to visit with the recommended specialist, Dr. Khizar Malik, the following week.

Going to a doctor who didn't know me and who hadn't been involved in my hospital treatment made me nervous; but, as I made my way around Celebration Hospital, I was too pleasantly distracted to notice. The hospital was a structurally pleasing building surrounded by the Disney community's wooded areas. Celebration Fitness—the gym in which I worked out—was actually set inside and owned by the hospital. Celebration Hospital was a comfortable place to go, and I felt more at ease walking through the familiar hallways than I would have anywhere else.

I arrived at Dr. Malik's office on the second floor and checked in. When my name was called, the nurse led me into the exam room, took my vitals, asked some general questions, and then had me wait for the doctor. The wait was brief, and Dr. Malik came in shortly after she'd left.

Dr. Malik was a soft-spoken man with a thick foreign accent, and I liked him from the start. He had ordered my MRI and other test results from Orlando Hospital, so he was aware of why I'd come to see him.

Dr. Malik discussed the results with me in detail and talked about my treatment options. As an MS specialist, he advised me to start taking MS medication in order to prevent or postpone another attack, to which I responded that I didn't want to inject unfamiliar medications into my system. That's when I discovered that I was blessed to have a doctor like Dr. Malik. Just like Dr. Nic, he was understanding and had a calming personality. He gave me packets of literature and told me to research the drugs he recommended: Rebif and Avonex. He hoped I would consider them, as he felt very strongly that I needed to start a medication regimen—just as strongly as I opposed the idea.

Once I got home, I immediately began studying the information in the packets and researching the drugs online. From what I read, it appeared that there were a great number of unappealing side effects and complications. Without sounding too much like a medical journal, I discovered that Rebif, a medication injected three times per week, would leave a patient with flu-like symptoms after each injection. The company's own website even stated that the exact way Rebif worked was not known. That was not reassuring at all.

Avonex, a similar type of drug, was to be injected once a week and would produce the same flu-like symptoms. Their website stated that the patient could potentially develop serious side effects, such as depression, mood disorders, allergic reactions, seizures, and liver, blood, thyroid, and heart problems. Was this for real?

During my investigation, I also read that most MS patients change medications periodically—after one loses its effectiveness, a new one has to be introduced in order to keep battling the symptoms. Through my best Sherlock Holmes medical investigation, I wasn't finding anything positive to go along with the bad news I'd discovered about Rebif and Avonex. Everything I read made me that much more unwilling to take the medication.

To me, it seemed like a complete waste of money to start taking ridiculously high-priced drugs that might *possibly* help me *somewhat* battle my disease, although no one could definitively explain how or guarantee that they would. That seemed absurd, and I wanted no part of that kind of system. I would just have to take my own path. What that was, I had no idea. I just knew it didn't include taking one MS medication after another.

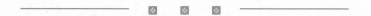

August rolled around, and I was just a few months removed from my hospitalization. I still didn't know my direction, where this disease was headed, or how I was going to fight it, but faith and prayer were keeping me sane. I reflected often on my time as a youth pastor at a small church in Fairhope, Alabama, and remembered the sermons I had given about God's plan for our lives. Now more than ever, I knew that this was a time in which I really needed to dig in and seek Him. Thank God I did, too, because with the end-of-summer heat, I would soon discover a new challenge regarding life with MS.

My wife and I were friends with two families from our community whose children were in school with ours. They were all planning to take a trip to Seaside, Florida, and, knowing what we had been through, they insisted we go along and take a break from the stress of the last few months.

For so many reasons, I didn't want to go. I didn't want to travel with my symptoms. I didn't want to socialize all that much. And, deep down, I knew what no one else did—that my marriage was a façade. For the sake of our children, though, I agreed to go.

Seaside is a beach community in the Florida panhandle known for its classic architecture, pastel-colored cottages, quaint shops, fine restaurants, art galleries, and amphitheatre entertainment. It's a lot like Celebration, but because it is on the Gulf Coast, it is known as a vacation hot spot for the wealthy. We searched online and found a three-story rental within walking distance of the beach and made the reservations.

As the trip grew closer, the kids got more and more excited. I, however, was dreading the seven-hour car ride, knowing that my wife would not likely help in the driving and that I would have to go the distance with the pain and numbness of my disease. Each day leading up to the trip, I worried about how I was going to make the drive and spend a week away from home, doctor, and hospital. As a result of my stress level, sleep, which had been a problem before, became almost impossible. It literally took everything in me not to cancel the trip.

The day we left was very difficult. My symptoms had not improved, and I was still experiencing a lack of coordination in my movements. I knew sitting in a car for seven hours would be horrendous, but I pushed the feelings aside, loaded up the car, and got into the driver's seat.

It was a cloudy day, and, as the three-car caravan drove northwest up I-10 toward Seaside, the clouds grew darker and darker. It was obvious that rain was in our forecast. About four hours into the trip, it began to thunder quite loudly as if the noise was right on top of the car. Soon those dark, ominous clouds opened up and unleashed a storm so strong that it was impossible to see out of the windows, even with the wipers on high. We all slowed down to a crawl and, with sparse cell phone reception, decided to pull over and wait it out. By the time we reached Seaside, our seven-hour drive had turned into an eleven-hour nightmare.

I'm not quite sure how I managed to drive that day with the MS difficulties, but I did. When we finally arrived at the beachside community, I got out of the car and tried to steady myself on the driveway pavement while my legs shook uncontrollably. My hands were both numb and in pain from holding the steering wheel for so long, and my back felt the same way down to my legs. I had an awful feeling that this was not going to be a fun week for me, and I was about to find out one of the main reasons why.

What I'd only aggravated to a degree at that point was the fact that multiple sclerosis is exasperated by heat. In what is called pseudo-exacerbation, its symptoms worsen in hot environments, intensifying pain, numbness, blurred vision, and fatigue. As MS patients, we have plaque on our nerves in the damaged places, which decreases the ability of our nerves to function. Apparently, heat only further slows down our nerve impulse transmissions in these areas.

Now, here I was—in Florida, in the middle of August, at the beach, spending a week outside in the sun. What was I thinking? We had a schedule filled with outdoor activities in the scorching sunshine, and, needless to say, I was not helping my MS condition by trying to play the hero and endure the experiences.

About halfway through the week, we decided to take a ride around the town on bicycle carriages in which the front riders would pedal and pull the others in a back carriage. We rented the bikes for an hour and pedaled our way through Seaside. Of course, I was one of the front riders.

As we moved along, I could feel my condition worsening. The seat constantly irritated my spine, and the continual pedaling movement churned my legs. Soon, I entered into a state of complete numbness and pain from the combination of physical exertion and heat. I must have been crazy, but I pushed myself to the end of the hour-long rental before going directly back to the house and virtually collapsing with exhaustion.

That was the epitome of my week's vacation. The adventures were painful and difficult. The fatigue was constant. The mental strain was unrelenting. When it was finally over, I drove as quickly as possible back to the security of my home and immediately made an appointment to see Dr. Malik to discuss how to handle this type of exacerbation.

——————————— ❖ ❖ ❖ ———————————

It took a week or so to get in to see Dr. Malik, and during the days of waiting I kept dwelling on what had happened in Seaside. I fixated on how difficult it had been to do simple things like ride a bike, load and unload a car, and even just sit and drive. I was eager to discuss all of this with the doctor and get his feedback on what was normal for an MS patient at this stage of the disease.

When I met with Dr. Malik, we spent a good amount of time chatting about the events of the trip and what had happened to me. When I asked him about the normalcy of my symptoms, his response was, "David, with multiple sclerosis, nothing is normal." He explained that everyone experiences similar symptoms but that they manifest differently for each patient. It all happens at different times with diverse ranges of severity and at varied stages of progression. Through Dr. Malik, I was learning that MS was so complex and wide-ranging in its behavior that no one actually knew why or how it happened, or, worse yet, how to treat it effectively. Generally speaking, MS is just an indescribable pain.

Dr. Malik also described the stages of MS. He felt that at this point, what I had was a form of relapsing-remitting MS, in which new symptoms appear in random attacks. But he also wasn't ruling out the idea that my MS might already be in the progressive stage and was slowly worsening over time. Because the attack was the first that I had acknowledged, it was just too soon to tell.

All this information was important to know, but it scared the heck out of me. Being hit in the face with everything being thrown at me made my thoughts spin in a thousand different directions, so much so that I couldn't even focus on which fear was going to get my attention. When I was finally able to concentrate on what I was being told, I heard Dr. Malik reiterate his belief that the best course of action would be for me to take some form of medication to hopefully slow down the progression. He shared what medications were available and how they could combat the pain, the spasticity of my muscles, and any feelings of helplessness or depression I would experience as a result. What I heard was that if I wanted to get through life with multiple sclerosis I had better resign myself to the use of a variety of drugs. And in my world that was just not happening.

I left Dr. Malik's office with a lot of head knowledge about MS, but I didn't feel like I had anything I could hold onto regarding how to deal with it. As I drove home, I found it difficult to process what I'd been told because of the many conflicting arguments going on between the voices in my head. I went back and forth between the fear surrounding my new reality—including the fact that I was now "disabled"—and my faith in God, that He would help me through this. Picture the old cartoon of the angel and the devil sitting on someone's shoulders. The angel was saying, "Yes, you can." The devil was saying, "No, you can't." And there I was with my head in the middle.

As I walked into my home, I felt the weight of dramatic life change. Inside, I had a sinking sensation that I was walking through the doorway of a prison.

I began devoting much of my time to searching for miracle cures online. During those days and weeks of fruitless investigation, I would often slip into believing that it was hopeless, and the devastation would overwhelm me. Conventional multiple sclerosis sites only led me to information about the different medications that were available, and it seemed to me that the known and possible side effects were still just not worth the chance. Holistic sites suggested certain supplements and special diets, but I couldn't wrap my head around the idea that if I stopped eating certain foods my MS would improve. Then there were the blog sites and the personal stories of MS patients. Reading how others were suffering, how depressed they were, and how they'd had to adapt their lifestyles to accommodate the disease only made me feel worse. The internet surfing was simply not helping me find out what I needed to do in order to beat this. Eventually, I decided to stop looking. I'd wasted enough time looking for answers in the wrong places and decided to look to the one source of wisdom in which I knew I could find truth: the Bible.

I began investigating God's Word when it came to healing, victory, and overcoming obstacles. Reading the truth of Scripture gave me hope and strength. Undoubtedly, there was a force out there that wanted to keep me down and defeated, and I knew that what I chose to believe would determine my fate.

Over time, my faith grew stronger as I was reminded that the Lord had a plan for me. His Word was the blueprint He had given me to follow, and the question then became what I was going to do with it. As someone who did not like to quit or lose, my gut instinct was to fight and to beat the disease; but everything I was hearing, seeing, and feeling from the outside was telling me to give up and not waste energy on a lost cause. I knew I shouldn't ask God, why me? But it was the inevitable question that kept haunting me. So I asked. And as I questioned God regarding His plan and why He had allowed this to happen to me, I kept getting the same answer: I would know in His time, not mine.

Chapter 3

GIVING UP

Living with multiple sclerosis became a daily roller coaster of symptoms and emotions. I had no control over my body, and I felt like I had no control of my life or mind. With my inability to focus on anything other than my disease, I no longer had any goals. My career as a television and film producer got shelved, and I lost my drive to be in shape. I was no longer connected to anything outside of myself. I didn't socialize, and, in many ways, I cut myself off from the outside world. Inside, I developed an attitude of self-pity as I tried to understand what was happening to my body. If I hadn't had my children and a connection to Christ, I know I would have checked out completely.

I did my best to get through the days and nights without losing my sanity. I continued to pray, read the Bible, go to church, and believe that God had a plan, but not knowing that plan was killing me. Because I had never been someone who openly shared his feelings, I kept every-thing inside and tried to handle it alone. I couldn't open up to my wife either, which made me feel even lonelier and more isolated. In order to make life tolerable, I pushed everything down and ignored it all as best I could. The highlights of my days were the interactions with my children. I couldn't wait for them to get home from school so I could shift my focus from my own situation to my love for them.

Helen and I had lost our emotional connection years before the MS had been diagnosed. Now that I was disabled, living together became an incredible strain. To me, it seemed like she was ignoring the reality of my incurable disease and the fact that many aspects of my daily life were unbearable for me. She didn't seem willing to comfort me or help me overcome any of the physical or psychological challenges. Instead, she lost herself in spending money, which only caused me more anxiety since I couldn't work. She even wanted to purchase and move into a bigger home. In light of our financial situation, I should have said no. It was the last thing I wanted to do. But I kept quiet and went along with the idea in order to keep the peace, believing it was going to be a big mistake.

This was my mode of operation in our broken marriage. In order to avoid confrontation, I let Helen do whatever she wanted, regardless of what I really felt or thought. Of course, I realize now that that was not the wise or godly way to do it, but I somehow always found a way to justify it at the time. The biggest reason I kept silent was because I feared our confrontations would lead to divorce, which I believed to be wrong, and I couldn't stomach the idea of leaving my children in that kind of situation.

I had been going to Dr. Malik on a monthly basis in order to monitor the MS, and, during our appointments, we also discussed what was going on with me mentally and emotionally. He was genuinely a good person and took the time to have conversations about more than just my disease. We talked about my marriage, and I confided in him about our unhappy situation. He commiserated with me, saying that having MS was hard enough to deal with without marital problems making it worse. Stress is a drain on a healthy person, but it can be devastating symptom-wise for someone with MS. Many patients take antidepressants to help them cope, so he asked if I wanted a prescription for one. Although I was sincerely stressed, I didn't want to start relying on drugs to get me through. I don't judge anyone who takes antidepressants, but it remained my personal choice not to start relying on chemicals. Instead, I told Dr. Malik that I would rely on my faith in Christ to sustain me. As a Muslim, he didn't quite see eye to eye with me, but he respected my beliefs.

During that visit, Dr. Malik ordered a new set of MRI tests in order to see what was happening with the lesions in my brain and spine. He explained that several things could have occurred: the lesions could have gotten smaller, which would help alleviate the symptoms; they could have stayed the same; or they could have grown. If the lesion near my optic nerve had worsened, the vision in my left eye would be at risk. If I had developed a lesion on my lower spine, I would partially or completely lose the mobility in my legs and eventually require a walker or a wheelchair, or, worse, become paralyzed from the waist down.

Over the past few months, I had noticed some new and different symptoms, so I was nervous about what the MRI would reveal. Because of my claustrophobia and my already heightened level of stress, I was once again prescribed Valium for the day of the test so that I would be able to handle the MRI enclosure. The morning of the test, I took two

Valium pills before I went to the hospital, and one as I entered the MRI room. They made sure I was as high as a kite so that I could handle lying in the machine for the full hour.

After a week of waiting, I went to see Dr. Malik again to discuss the results and look at my brain and spine. The tests showed that some of the lesions had expanded while the one by my optic nerve had gotten slightly smaller. The best news was that there were no new lesions, which meant that the MS had not progressed or worsened since my hospital stay. Unfortunately, this still hadn't changed the symptoms, nor did it guarantee anything positive was happening.

I left his office with a depressed and discouraged heart. I was going back to my horrible marriage, an indifference to my career, and to life with multiple sclerosis. On the short drive home, I prayed that Christ would heal me and put me back on a positive career path so that I could once again have a way of supporting my family and burying my marital problems. If only I could be physically whole again, I thought I could handle the marriage. But no instant healing ever came, and I continued to walk down a road of personal darkness.

Weeks went by without an income, and I continued dealing with my fluctuating MS symptoms, all the while looking for a new house I didn't want. Prior to my diagnosis, I had been a highly motivated person who always found ways to bring in money, but my mindset had shifted, and I started feeling like life was not worth living. I occupied my time by taking my kids to and from school, trying to avoid interaction with Helen, and fighting the fatigue and foggy thinking that came with the disease. Depression set in, yet I denied being depressed. I put on a good show so that I wouldn't concern my children, but it was becoming more and more difficult to put up a front.

Eventually we found a house and prepared to relocate. It was a move that went against everything I believed to be right, but I didn't have the energy to fight. We would use our current home as an income-producing rental property in order to cover the monthly mortgage, taxes, and expenses. Little did we know that the real estate market was about to take a nosedive and that property values would plummet.

That, however, was exactly what happened. Our rental home couldn't demand the typical high fees of Celebration, and our new home ended up being worth almost $200,000 less than we had invested in it. The cash drain had opened up like a well, and money poured through it rapidly. Don't ask me how we managed to go on a $10,000 vacation to Breckenridge, Colorado, and a $5,000 Disney cruise, but we did. The kids had no idea we were going down a hole with no way out, and Helen just didn't seem to be getting it, living in perpetual denial.

The subject of divorce had come up many times, but I still didn't want to do it. Now, with the additional factor of my having MS, that avenue didn't look like it would have a positive outcome for any of us, so I hung in there—until I couldn't any longer. I prayed over and over for God's direction. I knew that the Lord didn't condone divorce and that marriage held an unbreakable bond, and I wrestled and agonized over the decision for weeks. The only conclusion I could come to was that God's forgiveness remains a mystery. Even when we fall short, He still offers us His love and grace. During that time in my life, His forgiveness became more valuable to me than I can ever express. The end of our marriage was on its way.

Every day I wondered what God's plan was for me in my condition and what the eventual outcome would be. Moments of depression, anxiety, and defeat were often followed by glimpses of strength, hope, and purpose, and of trusting the Lord for His direction. His faithfulness remained clear, and He would always give me something to hang on to—something that seemed "coincidental" but that I knew could only come from Him. Those occurrences kept me going. They were small miracles that showed me He was still with me and that He was working on my behalf.

One of these miracles came in the form of a God-orchestrated connection. Many days, while dropping my kids off at school, I would see a man who had a son in Dean's grade who also seemed to be struggling with movement. He fought to get in and out of his Range Rover and used a walker to get around. I always wondered about his condition since he looked healthy despite his uncoordinated, shaky movements. I'd never spoken to him, but I'd heard many people ask him how he was feeling.

I didn't think much of it until that man wound up being my new neighbor after we moved. His name was Phil, and he and his family had lived in the house next to ours for many years. Shortly after we moved in, Phil and his wife, Debbie, came over to introduce themselves and welcome us to the neighborhood.

Phil and I hit it off right away, and we began to talk about who we were, what we did, and life in general. Without my even having to ask, Phil told me that he had multiple sclerosis. I was in shock! What were the odds that my neighbor—a man my age—would have MS? The first thing that came to my mind was that God obviously had a purpose. This was a clear indication that, for whatever reason, God had led us to purchase the home next to Phil's. Even if I hadn't agreed with the decision to buy a new house, I was grateful that there was a blessing involved.

As the weeks and months went by, Phil and I became close friends, and we spent many hours together discussing our lives and our disease. After a twenty-five-year battle against MS, Phil had really started struggling both physically and emotionally. The long fight had taken its toll on him.

Phil had once been a very successful builder in the central Florida area, even winning design awards for his construction. He had worked long, hard hours and reaped the financial rewards. And Phil had also been an athlete. Based on his build, it was obvious that he had been in great shape before the MS had ravaged him. During our chats, Phil would tell me stories about how he had played football when he was younger, and he emphasized how difficult life had become after he'd lost the ability to do what he once could.

I watched as Phil spastically maneuvered himself with his walker, struggled to find his thoughts in our conversations, and constantly rubbed his legs to combat the pain. On his worst days, which became increasingly more frequent, he used a wheelchair to get around and needed more assistance. Because of the severity of his condition, Phil was taking many medications for pain, depression, and the MS symptoms, and he would alter his meds from one MS drug to another trying to find one that would stop the progression. He even went so far as to get monthly chemotherapy treatments, since it was believed that they helped stop and even reverse the disease. But nothing seemed to help, and Phil was getting worse fast.

Phil was honest about his depression, and he told me how he thought life with a disability was, quite frankly, terrible. In some ways I felt guilty for not being afflicted to his degree and for being able to walk without assistance. Seeing Phil's condition also scared me and made me wonder if that would someday—any day—be me.

That thought haunted me constantly. I smiled and stayed positive around Phil because I didn't want to add to his depression by complaining and expressing my own hopelessness. In my spirit, I sensed the Lord asking me to be strong and courageous for my friend, but when I was alone in my own home, I couldn't keep from seeing myself in Phil's shoes. Time after time, I dropped to my knees and prayed until my prayers became a mess of pleading, crying, bargaining, and accepting.

"Please, Lord, not me," I would pray. "Don't let me end up like Phil. Heal me."

Then it would be, "Lord, show me the purpose in this trial. I know there is a reason. Use me for your will."

Finally, I would revert to bargaining with God, telling Him that, if He healed me, I would do whatever He wanted. But nothing changed. I had multiple sclerosis, and all my pleading and pseudo-acceptance of what I knew God had allowed in my life wouldn't change it. I was distraught and unhappy. I wanted a way out—a way to escape my fate. I had no idea what would make me strong enough to continue a life of battling MS, but I knew that my life as it stood was not the way.

In September of 2007, my life did change, but it wasn't in the way I'd been hoping for. In a stream of events that would make for a great Hollywood film like *War of the Roses*, my marriage finally imploded. Helen and I decided to stop playing games and faking the idea that we were a team. Truly, I believed there was nothing I could do to keep the marriage intact.

Let me be clear: I do not condone divorce. I know from experience that it is destructive and devastating. Through Christ alone I had kept it together for fifteen years; but, between the stress of coping with MS and the hollowness of a marriage that lacked any connection, I felt like there were no more options. I packed my bags and moved into the vacant townhouse we owned down the road. With Florida's speedy divorce process, it didn't take long before our marriage was ended.

Chapter 4

THE BATTLE BEGINS

After the divorce I constantly fought the depressing fact that I was no longer in the same home as my children. Despite my strained relationship with Helen, I spent many days each week going back to my old home to spend time with them. It was a strange and uncomfortable situation for everyone, but the kids needed me, and I very much needed them. Every Wednesday and every other weekend, Deric, Anna, and Dean would also come stay with me at the townhouse. I knew they would rather have been in their own rooms at their house, but that was just how it had to be now that we were a split family.

In order to generate some income, I traded stocks during the day as I tried to decide my next career move. With all the changes going on in my life, though, that was tremendously difficult. It was hard to think clearly at all. Between fighting depression, adjusting to my new role as a single dad, and dealing with MS, life was a mess, and the stress only made the MS symptoms worse, almost unbearable. I spent a great deal of time going to doctors to try to manage what was happening to my body, while at night I would lie in bed alone, missing my children and praying for answers from God. The Bible became my refuge as I read the Lord's Word and escaped into the truth of Scripture.

> He gives strength to the weary and increases the power of the weak. (Isa. 40:29)

> Surely God is my salvation; I will trust and not be afraid. The LORD, the LORD, is my strength and my song; he has become my salvation. (Isa. 12:2)

> My soul is weary with sorrow; strengthen me according to your word. (Ps. 119:28)

While seeking the Lord's direction, I particularly prayed for wisdom in several areas, as there were just a few things I needed to figure out. First, how was I going to fight this disease? Second, was sitting at home staring at the stock market all day what I wanted to do for the rest of my life, or should I try to get back into creating entertainment? Finally, did I want to stay single or should I look for a woman with whom I could potentially share the rest of my life?

With the computer as my new best friend, I slowly started to explore my options in the relationship area. And I reiterate the word *slowly*. Because of my lack of motivation and my fears of being rejected because of MS, my confidence was on the fence. During my first month on my own, I had become sort of a recluse, doing very little other than going to the grocery store and seeing my kids. The MS had given me a noticeable limp, and I was now dragging my left leg everywhere I went. That entire side of my body was still experiencing most of the effects from the MS attack, and it had suffered more permanent damage than my right side. I was embarrassed to be seen at all.

And, to knock my pride down one more notch, I was now driving an old, beat-up van that was loaned to me from my soon-to-be former sister-in-law's boyfriend. I had driven a new Mercedes-Benz every few years since my mid-twenties, and I was accustomed to that kind of luxury and prestige. Now, I was picking my kids up from school in a hunk of junk. I know it embarrassed them too, since their mom was still taking them in her Mercedes GL luxury SUV. This was Celebration: the Disney community in which dreams came true and everyone was successful. You just didn't drive an old, run-down van in Celebration. That was for the people who lived outside our fair boundaries. It was a prideful attitude, but it was the sentiment of those who lived there.

Don't get me wrong, I loved living in Celebration. It was a beautiful city within a city, and it was where I had met some of the nicest people. Now, however, I was starting to see that the overall image was based on a cloud of arrogance.

With life continuing on much the same as it had, I continued to endure many sleepless nights. While lying awake, I would contemplate my life, where I was now and what had happened to me. I thought long and hard about my new state of humility. I looked for purpose now, and I questioned everything. To that point, I had given to many in need, helped struggling family members, and had faithfully contributed to the churches I'd attended over the years. But now I questioned my motivation in life. Was I more excited about the money I made or the people I helped? Was I more proud of my accomplishments or more thankful to the Lord for blessing me the way He had? I began to second-guess my motives and check my pride.

It's ironic how when you are convinced that you have everything you set out to reach in life, the Lord shows you the truth. For me, happiness had been tied to my success in business and not to the most important aspects of life. Of course, my children were the exception to this, and I loved them with all of my heart. But I had focused on material things in the other areas of my life. In many ways, I praised God externally but internally worshipped man-made things. In my current state, I came to the conclusion that I wasn't doing what I really felt God wanted of me. I was lost, floundering in an existence that contradicted everything my soul truly wanted. Now, in a pivotal new season of life, it was time to re-evaluate my purpose, my goals, and my direction.

Every day I read the Bible, prayed, and searched my soul. Slowly I began to emerge from my cocoon and started to incorporate a few routine activities into my life again so that I could establish a feeling of normalcy.

My first action from this positive line of thinking was to get back into the gym. Of course, there were many obstacles to face stemming from impaired coordination, a dwindled body, and the remaining numbness and pain; but, if I wanted to stay sane, I knew I needed to push myself beyond what was now my comfort zone.

I was still a member at the Fitness Centre inside Celebration Hospital; I just hadn't used it since I'd been diagnosed with MS. The gym was within minutes of my home, even walking distance if I was healthy, so I began planning out a strategy. I had to determine how I could best avoid being noticed by neighbors or embarrassed when strangers saw me holding onto machines to steady myself. If I trained early enough—maybe when the gym opened at 5:30 a.m.—no one would be there. Because the gym was multileveled and expansive, there would be plenty of places to hide from the other members, especially if only a few were there.

I was motivated. I drove to the gym that next Monday, pushing myself to get out of bed before the sun came up in order to work out. I was nervous about going, but the Lord helped me push through and stick to the plan. And what I soon discovered was that dealing with the emotions and fears that came from going to the gym that day would prove to be transformational.

I approached the doors to the gym with such anxiety. *Would I be able to do what I had planned? Would others see me as strange or disabled? What if I couldn't stick with the training?* I truly needed the Lord's hand to push me inside.

I walked into the workout area wearing a headset blaring loud classic rock music, which put me into my own world. The place was like a ghost town. To say there were ten people in there would have been an overstatement. And they were so spread out from each other that I would have had to intentionally run into someone in order to get interaction.

It was great. I felt like I had the huge gym all to myself. I could fall over and no one would see or care, which was exactly what I had wanted. I thanked God.

One thing I didn't expect was that even with my many years as a gym owner, boxer, and bodybuilder, I felt strangely lost among the weights and machines. My body had become used to being inactive since my diagnosis, which by now had been more than a year ago. I worked out slowly, using very light weights and doing small movements. It was difficult to maneuver around and get in and out of the equipment, and I could barely hold on to the bars and weights with my left hand.

The movements caused me pain and intensified the tingling throughout my body, but I didn't care. I was working out!

I continued to go to the gym four days every week, even though the motions heightened my MS symptoms. It just felt good to move and use my body again. I felt alive and strong. It was like I was doing something to counter the disease—taking the control back from the MS instead of letting it dominate me and determine my course.

Working out again was just one of the small steps that helped me eventually regain my life. I began dating periodically and socializing more in an effort to re-enter the world. Granted, it was a different world now that I was an MS patient, but it was a world outside the walls of my home—and I needed to live in it.

***

My first holiday season alone was just around the corner, and I wasn't looking forward to it. I saw them as lonely days without my children. I'd never missed a birthday, holiday, or any event with them for that matter, so I knew this was going to be a rough end to the year.

Thanksgiving was an awkward occasion. My children wanted me to come to their house for dinner, and Helen thought it would be a good idea as well since this was the first holiday after the split. At the time, the divorce was still in process, so I spent Thanksgiving with my children and my soon-to-be ex-wife.

I was reluctant to commit and knew the day would be uncomfortable, but the prodding of my kids influenced me to go. As I expected, the evening was filled with uneasy conversation and painful silences. That was the last holiday we spent together as a broken family.

***

Before being diagnosed with MS, I had made friends with a neighboring couple—John and Jennifer—who had two children, one of whom was in class with Anna at Celebration Elementary. John was a Florida state trooper and a bodybuilder, and Jennifer was also a bodybuilder who was doing quite well in her forties as a competitive amateur. We'd hit it off right away after meeting and had much to talk about between training, dieting, and our kids. To that point, though, we hadn't had much chance to socialize, since John worked mostly at nights and slept during the days. Even so, we managed to find some times to hang out and let our kids play together.

John and Jennifer had been very encouraging when they'd found out about my diagnosis. John would often stop by in his patrol car on his way to or from work and talk to me about working out. He could tell I was hesitant about training beyond my current level, but he seemed to think it would be a good idea for me to get back into a hard-core bodybuilding gym. He told me about his workouts with his training partner, Darren Barnes, who was a certified fitness trainer, an amateur competitive bodybuilder, and the manager of a bodybuilding gym. My conversations with John made me think about how much I missed training like that and how I hated not being as big as I was before MS, or even in my twenties for that matter. In my past, I had lived for bodybuilding. I'd owned gyms, trained friends, and thrown myself into intense workouts that would almost make me vomit. Even now I wanted to travel back to the eighties—a time in which I was one of the big, strong bodybuilders who intimidated the gym crowds. But here I was at age forty-eight, almost forty-nine, and suffering from an incurable neurological disease.

John didn't want to hear it. He kept hinting that maybe I should go to the gym—a real bodybuilding gym instead of a luxury fitness center—and work out with him and Darren. I thought to myself, *Is John crazy? How could I train with guys like that and keep up with them?* I was embarrassed just thinking about going to a gym filled with body-builders. No way did I want them to see me having trouble moving and struggling to lift light weights. I'd just stick to the hospital fitness center. At least if I hurt myself or had an MS attack I would be in the right place.

◈   ◈   ◈

It was the last week of November 2007. I had been going to the fitness center consistently for a while now, and John knew it. One day he showed up at my front door, ready to go to the gym and train with Darren, and instructed me to get my workout clothes on and get in his car. Obviously I didn't want to do what he asked, but John was a big, powerful guy—a very strong-willed man and a cop. If he'd had the desire, he could have easily picked me up, thrown me into the car, and forced me to go. I got ready—quickly—and went with him. And though I never would have admitted it to him, I was glad he was doing it, even if I was scared to death to take on the hardcore environment.

When we got to the gym, Darren, who was the gym's manager, was already waiting for us. John had planned everything all along and had told Darren that I would be training with them. Suddenly, after years of being a leader in the gym, I now found myself following the lead of other training partners.

Neither John nor Darren felt the need to ease up on their own routines, but they were extremely patient and helpful in getting me through mine. My biggest challenge that day was fatigue. I tried to keep up the pace, but it was evident that I was struggling to get past this first workout, and the guys knew it. They witnessed my coordination difficulty and my inability to securely grasp the weights. It had been a long time since I'd pushed myself this hard, and I was really feeling the pain and other symptoms of the disease.

But I wasn't about to stop training that day. Despite the stumbling blocks I was creating in their normal workout routines, John and Darren stood by me and encouraged me through it. And the sense of accomplishment I felt when we finished was astounding. There was no doubt in my mind or heart that I would become a bodybuilder again.

As John and I drove home, we talked about the workout. John made it a point to say he'd told me so—he'd told me I could do it. "You're a strong guy," he said. "You're a bodybuilder, and you will always be one. You have to train any way you can, and you have to beat this disease."

Looking back, I can honestly say that if it wasn't for John's belief in me and his persistence in getting me to the gym, I don't think I would ever have resumed bodybuilding. Sure, I was getting to the fitness center at the hospital and doing light, easy movements, but on my own, with no encouragement from a guy like John, I doubt I would ever have had the courage to get back into a bodybuilding environment.

According to John, Darren had said it was okay with him if I wanted to keep training with them, which I did. He gave me a weekly workout schedule and began picking me up each training day. Now, not only was I blessed with two extraordinary training partners, I also had a chauffeur. Not a bad deal.

On December 10, 2007, I entered my third week of working out with John and Darren. We trained four days a week, taking Wednesdays, Saturdays, and Sundays off. My forty-ninth birthday fell on a Monday—a training day.

I awakened to sunlight coming in through the blinds and lay in bed listening to the lonely silence in the room. There were no children jumping on the bed, no cards, no cake, and no one to sing "Happy Birthday" to me. I was alone, and all I had to hold onto were the memories of birthdays in the past when my children had been constantly by my side.

Being separated from Deric, Anna, and Dean was hands down the worst part of my situation, even more devastating than the fact that I had worked for more than thirty years and had almost nothing left to show for it. So, on this first day of my last year before turning fifty, I remained in bed alone feeling the numbness, tightness, and pins and needles that were constantly in my arms and legs as a result of MS.

When I looked to the side, all I could see was darkness, as if a black hole had taken over the vision in my left eye. Now, my thoughts were a cloud of lost names and sentences without words. I searched my mind for traces of thoughts I'd once been able to think without effort, but struggled to find them. My body was unrecognizable to me, and I was nothing like the man I'd been just a short year and a half ago.

As I lay there contemplating my life, I found it hard to accept the fact that this was who I was at this stage of my life. After almost half a century of hard work, I felt defeated. The silence in the room magnified the emptiness and filled me with despair. I looked around my new, temporary home and longed to have the birthday dinner, the cake, and my children serenading me, but I knew that wasn't coming this year. My forty-ninth birthday celebrated a life that had been torn from me in so many ways.

I kept saying to myself, *This is not happening to me.* I closed my eyes and prayed that everything I'd once had would reappear right in front of me again. I wanted to wake up one day to realize that this had all been just a terrible nightmare that had lasted a little too long. I wanted to open my eyes and have my health, my possessions, my business, and my children back. That would have been heaven. But this was no nightmare. This was reality. And it was a reality I did not want.

I was alone with nothing but a body that had decided to no longer cooperate and a mind that found it hard to grasp simple thoughts. That morning in particular, I found myself swimming desperately in the whirlpool I called life, and thought to myself, *Now what?*

I got out of bed and walked to the mirror. The reflection staring back at me seemed foreign. It wasn't me. It was a forty-nine-year-old man with an incurable disease who was struggling to finish light workouts at the gym.

What had happened to the Dave who had endless energy? Where was the guy who had once pushed himself so hard in the gym that he'd been able to bend bars? That twenty-year-old athlete was still in there somewhere; I just knew it. There had to be something I could do to save my body and reach back inside to that powerful, motivated Dave.

It was clear that I had a choice: I could put on my armor, grab my shield and spear, and fight this battle like a warrior, or I could lay my weapons down and let the enemy ravage me. I grabbed my Bible and read Ephesians 6:10–20, putting myself in Paul's shoes:

> Finally, be strong in the Lord and in his mighty power.
> Put on the full armor of God, so that you can take your
> stand against the devil's schemes. For our struggle is not
> against flesh and blood, but against the rulers, against
> the authorities, against the powers of this dark world and
> against the spiritual forces of evil in the heavenly realms.
> Therefore put on the full armor of God, so that when the
> day of evil comes, you may be able to stand your ground,
> and after you have done everything, to stand. Stand firm
> then, with the belt of truth buckled around your waist,
> with the breastplate of righteousness in place, and with
> your feet fitted with the readiness that comes from the
> gospel of peace. In addition to all this, take up the shield

of faith, with which you can extinguish all the flaming
arrows of the evil one. Take the helmet of salvation and
the sword of the Spirit, which is the word of God.

 And pray in the Spirit on all occasions with all kinds
of prayers and requests. With this in mind, be alert and
always keep on praying for all the Lord's people. Pray also
for me, that whenever I speak, words may be given me
so that I will fearlessly make known the mystery of the
gospel, for which I am an ambassador in chains. Pray that
I may declare it fearlessly, as I should.

Some contend that Paul wrote the book of Ephesians while he was a
prisoner in the city of Rome. It is also believed that his afflictions contributed to his great appreciation for the things of God. Paul's tribulations were great; but it seemed to me that his spiritual experiences and
God's comfort were even greater, and it encouraged me to find strength
in my own challenge.

 So with God's Word as my guide, I chose to fight, and I prayed
for His power to work inside me as I battled this enemy. That day—
December 10, 2007, my forty-ninth birthday—I resolved to undertake
a challenge that would push my mind, body, and spirit to their limits.
It would mark the beginning of my journey to a place where few had
ventured and to accomplish what no one my age with multiple sclerosis
had ever attempted.

 I had a plan.

Chapter 5

THE CHALLENGE IS BORN

Today was the day. My life was going to take a different path. In my mind, I wasn't an MS patient anymore; I was a man who had the goal of beating the odds and overcoming the disease.

That morning, in the middle of my despair and loneliness, I decided to take on the incredible, odds-defying challenge of competing in a high level amateur bodybuilding contest, which no one with MS had ever done at my age. I didn't plan to enter the disabled division, either. I would stand onstage next to the healthy athletes and compete against them without any special considerations.

It had been more than twenty-five years since I'd stepped onto a bodybuilding contest stage, and I hadn't trained like a competitive bodybuilder for at least fifteen, even before my MS diagnosis. Even if I was healthy, I knew I wouldn't be anywhere near the condition of today's amateur National Physique Committee (NPC) bodybuilders. With all of the advancements that had been made in the areas of diet and training, coupled with the complexity of performance-enhancing drugs and supplements, amateur bodybuilding had been taken to a new level—one that far surpassed the pros of my day. But, to me, it wouldn't be about winning. It would be a personal challenge to not give up on life.

⁂

As I waited for John to pick me up, I felt a new sense of commitment. I climbed into his car and told him that I had an idea about how to fight MS, and he was eager to hear it. When I told him what I was going to do he wasn't as shocked as I thought he would be. "If anyone can do this, you can," he said.

We went to the gym and trained with Darren, but I didn't tell him right away because I wanted to talk to him in greater detail. I knew that in order to do this successfully I would need more than just training partners; I would need a trainer who could spend time developing a specific bodybuilding routine and diet for me to follow. It just seemed natural for me to ask Darren, since he had been training with me for several weeks and knew what I was going through. He also was a certified fitness trainer working with winning amateur competitive bodybuilders and was a top-three-ranked competitive bodybuilder himself. Plus, he was just a great guy.

When we finished training, I asked Darren if he could meet me at my home later that evening. This wasn't an easy question with a simple answer. It would require a huge commitment on his part, and I needed some time to figure out how to ask him.

That evening when Darren arrived at my home, I sat him down in my office and looked him in the eye. I could tell that he was wondering what was up, so I didn't prolong the conversation. Without beating around the bush, I explained my entire plan and philosophy to him and expressed my passion to complete the challenge.

Darren's response was a little different than John's.

"This is crazy," he said. "Are you sure you want to do this?"

There was a long moment of silence, and it was obvious that the wheels were turning in his head. After the pause, he announced his verdict.

"I'm in," he said. "I'll go home and work on a diet and your training routine. When do you want to start?"

I smiled at him. "Tomorrow."

This would be a massive undertaking for Darren, and there had to be a starting point with a slow progression to my—or I should say *our*—goal. During the first month or two, we would work on building a training base that would prepare my body for much more grueling workouts. I'd also start maintaining a strict diet to put on some much-needed muscle. John would continue training with us, but our focus would shift to getting me ready to compete. Darren was currently competing, so he was already in that groove. Between his guidance and John's encouragement, I had the perfect combination of knowledge and motivation behind me.

As the training days started to peel away from the calendar, I became increasingly inspired. I knew in my heart that there was a God-given purpose in all of this. The disease, my personal losses, the new refusal to give up on life, and, now, my goal to complete this odds-defying task were what I believed to be the Lord's way of showing me something bigger than what I had been seeing—a greater vision with a broader perspective. This wasn't just about physical strength; it was about God's glory and about His power being made perfect in my weakness (2 Cor. 12:9).

I was finally understanding the point, and I was determined to follow the path He'd laid out for me and to see where it would lead.

In looking for ways to facilitate His strength inside me, I constantly searched for verses of Scripture that would reinforce the point of my journey. I found plenty of them.

> Not that I have already obtained all this, or have already arrived at my goal, but I press on to take hold of that for which Christ Jesus took hold of me. (Phil. 3:12)

> I press on toward the goal to win the prize for which God has called me heavenward in Christ Jesus. (Phil. 3:14)

> So we make it our goal to please him, whether we are at home in the body or away from it. (2 Cor. 5:9)

Soon, after a short time of studying goal-oriented Scripture, it also started to sink in that this drive I had—to stand on a bodybuilding stage despite MS—would also be about impacting others for Christ. I could be an example of how faith and the strength and the power of God through Jesus could move mountains—or simply rebuild muscles in the face of disease.

> My goal is that they may be encouraged in heart and united in love, so that they may have the full riches of complete understanding, in order that they may know the mystery of God, namely, Christ. (Col. 2:2)

> The goal of this command is love, which comes from a pure heart and a good conscience and a sincere faith. (1 Tim. 1:5)

It was now January 2008, and, with the new year, my direction was getting more vivid. It was time to put a clear plan into action and to give it a name. The title came quickly: the MS Bodybuilding Challenge. It was a simple yet powerful way to capture the nature of the test.

During my next meeting with Darren, we began to talk about strategy in greater detail. I knew I couldn't do this alone and that it would take a team of professionals, including a sports doctor, a nutritional supplement company, and others. As a competitor, Darren was already connected to supplement providers, so he reached out to his contacts while I started looking for doctors.

I started investigating sports medicine doctors in the area and, through an online search, found Dr. Brad Homan, D.O., who was the chief of surgery and director of sports medicine at Florida Hospital Celebration Health. He was also the medical director of the hospital's fitness center where I'd previously trained. I sent him an introductory email explaining what I was trying to accomplish, and within a day he called me.

As an athlete and bodybuilder himself, Dr. Homan understood what I wanted to achieve. Although he knew it would be a difficult task for a man with MS who was quickly approaching age fifty, he was willing to help; so we scheduled an appointment to go over details.

After our second meeting, Dr. Homan agreed to monitor my health free of charge to make sure I was training properly and that my blood levels were in range. This was a huge blessing, as I also discovered that Dr. Homan had an incredible resume. He was the team physician for the Orlando Sharks professional indoor soccer team, a staff physician for the TNA professional wrestling company, the sports medicine director and practice coverage doctor for the NBA pre-draft combine, and a staff physician at the Coach Tom Shaw performance enhancement camp at

Disney's Wide World of Sports. Clearly God had dropped the perfect doctor right into my lap.

While I was out "finding" the sports doctor, Darren was out speaking with the owner of the Orlando Max Muscle franchise, a local branch of the national supplement company. When he returned from his meeting, Darren shared the good news that Orlando Max Muscle was willing to supply all of my supplements leading into my first contest.

The very next day, I went to the store to meet Ram, the owner, and to fill up my car with everything from protein powder to multivitamins—all at no cost. Ram was just excited to see how far I could go while utilizing the Max Muscle products. His support shocked and elated me, and I knew that we were on the right track. With the supplements and Darren's training routine, I'd be able to pack on the muscle. I was pumped—or, at least, I would be soon!

In a surprising side-effect, I discovered that the excitement of moving forward in one area of my life spilled over into other aspects as well. I was motivated, enthusiastic, and more energetic despite the MS. It was a new chapter—one filled with hope and the belief that all things were possible with Christ.

In my study of Scripture, I searched the book of Job. Here was a man who had dealt with difficulties and suffered greatly yet had never lost sight of who he was in God's eyes, nor had he blamed God for what happened to him (Job 1:21–22). Even though he lost everything, from possessions to health to loved ones, he remained faithful to the Lord and persevered to receive a blessing in the end. To me, if Job could overcome those overwhelming afflictions and remain strong in his faith, I could overcome living with MS and starting life over at age fifty—or close to it.

It was time for me to move on, keep my faith in God firm, and reach out to Him for guidance and strength. In His power, I stayed faithful to the training plan and diet and gained strength with each new day.

This spurred me on to take leaps in my personal life, as well. I knew I had to have a balance between this new goal and life outside bodybuilding and the gym. It was time to meet new people and diversify my interests so that I didn't get lost in my drive to compete in a bodybuilding contest.

As in all competitive sports, bodybuilding can become an obsession and not just a goal. I'd both seen and experienced it in the past. Competitors begin to eat, sleep, and think the sport 24/7 and ignore the rest of life. I didn't want that to happen to me. So with my divorce final, I ventured into the world of online dating.

Certainly, I could write a book on that adventure alone. After what had previously taken place in my marriage, I found that I struggled to trust women and feared repeating the mistakes of my past; so I proceeded cautiously. I went on a few dates with women I met, and I made a few friends, but no romance was sparked. It was clear that I was more focused on figuring out life than finding a mate, so I decided to call it quits.

The experience, however, was a step in the right direction, as it had helped me achieve the balance I'd desired and allowed me to break from concentrating on the MS Bodybuilding Challenge. With the competition drawing nearer by the day, though, and my desire to show the world what God could do with an MS-stricken man, I decided to put the pursuit of a serious relationship on the shelf.

One aspect of life that couldn't be ignored, however, was the need for income. In prayer I asked the Lord to open doors and guide my steps as

I re-entered the business world. This was not going to be easy. In fact, I often wondered which was more challenging: rebuilding my body or my life.

It was so difficult to balance my days. I knew what I needed to accomplish in the various aspects of the journey, but the list was overwhelming and, at times, hard to swallow. Daily I battled the thoughts that would tell me I couldn't accomplish my goals. The voice of defeat constantly whispered that this mountain was too high to climb.

But I was also being really hard on myself. I wasn't even considering the fact that I had just suffered three of the most devastating tragedies in life: a health crisis, a divorce, and the halt of my business. My mind oscillated like a fan, stirring everything up and constantly revolving around giving up and giving it all to God.

What I was going through was no small trial; it was a giant of a task. I felt like I was David fighting three Goliaths. All I could do was take one day at a time and keep telling myself that the Lord would never put more on my shoulders than I could handle. Even so, I kept crying out to Him asking, "How strong do you think these shoulders are, Lord?"

Every day I would read the Bible and pray. I interacted with my children either in person or by phone, worked out at the gym, and ate the six meals, protein drinks, and supplements Darren had assigned in my diet plan. I looked for opportunities in the stock market, and I did my best to manage my MS symptoms. Weekly, I did domestic chores, talked to my parents, did something fun with my kids, and tried to socialize. The rest of the time was spent working with Darren to organize the MS Bodybuilding Challenge and trying to find what was next for me in business.

The stock market income was sporadic, and I needed to find something that I could count on each week in order to keep what little I had left intact. Plus, I wanted to do something I was excited to do, and that was not trading stocks. The only profession that had generated that kind of passion inside me, other than when I had owned fitness centers, had been the entertainment industry.

I'd been in touch with Mark Simon—the animation producer who'd helped me with the *Creepers* project—and his wife Jeanne. Over the years we had developed a friendship, and, prior to the divorce, my younger children, Anna and Dean, had been friends with the Simons' twin boys. Even after the divorce, I would occasionally go to their home for dinner, and we would discuss projects they were working on.

During our visits, Mark and Jeanne encouraged me to work with them and get back into the TV and film business. The Simons were entrepreneurs in every sense of the word and were both very success-driven. Mark worked many hours on his animation company while simultaneously building their newest business enterprise. Jeanne handled much of the creative writing and took care of their boys. During their years in the entertainment industry, the Simons had accumulated many credits, and novice producers and concept creators considered them to be experts in the field.

With this reputation, they'd developed a business that involved training others how to be successful in the industry. Mark and Jeanne felt I would be a natural to work with them in this venture. With my sales and business experience and the quick success I'd had in creating and pitching both *Creepers* and two sports competition shows to FOX Sports, Mark and Jeanne believed I could be an asset to their team. Because I trusted them and enjoyed them both as friends, I agreed to help them in the company sales.

Going in, we all knew this would be a temporary situation, as I was hoping to regenerate my own company, Lyons Entertainment, which had been sidetracked after the MS diagnosis. And I didn't have to wait long for an opportunity. Not long after joining the Simons, I was approached by Berchman Richard, the creator and co-owner of a production company, who asked me to become the producer and host of their motorcycle show *Hog Heaven*. Berchman had seen me speak at one of the Simons' seminars and was impressed enough to contact me. I accepted his offer and moved forward one more step.

With all of the life rebuilding taking place, I maintained a sharp focus on the MS Bodybuilding Challenge and kept spreading the word about what I was doing. With a great trainer, a sports medicine doctor, and a nutritional supplement company on my team, I wanted to let the entire bodybuilding and fitness world know about my challenge. It was my deepest desire to show the world that through faith anyone could overcome even the most incredible odds.

I began emailing everyone I could think of who might care about my undertaking, while Darren reached out to others. He spoke to his boss and secured a complimentary membership for me at his gym and shared the news about what he and I were doing together. In a huge response, it seemed like everyone at the gym was behind me, including retired pro football star Greg Favors and NWA pro wrestler Raul Paoli (a.k.a. Red Skull), both of whom worked out at the facility. Everyone wanted to see me standing on that contest stage someday.

In response to my emails, I began receiving notes of support from people across the country. One came from former professional bodybuilder Ed Corney, who had competed into his late sixties and was now in his seventies. Ed had been one of the top competitors in his day and had been one of Arnold Schwarzenegger's training partners, as well as one of the stars of the 1977 documentary *Pumping Iron*. For me, getting an email from Ed was like getting a letter from the president. I felt honored that Ed, in his retirement, would care enough to respond to someone he'd never met and even cheer him on.

My next email came from the director of country music star Clay Walker's multiple sclerosis charity, Band Against MS (BAMS). The organization, which had been established in 2003, provided educational information for those living with MS, funded programs that researched cures, and facilitated others aimed at helping those with the disease. Walker, who had been diagnosed with MS in 1996, wanted to help others in his situation, and the director's email stated that the singer himself and the BAMS organization were in support of my challenge.

Over the years, my heart to touch lives for Christ had always been strong. I'd been a youth pastor at a small church in Alabama in the late nineties and participated in my good friend Pastor Neil Kennedy's ministries and youth programs whenever I could. Now I wanted to align the MS Bodybuilding Challenge with my faith in a public way.

Other supporters continued to surface. From companies to individuals, the responses fueled me on and gave me incredible motivation and drive. One of the connections dearest to me stemmed from the Fellowship of Christian Athletes (FCA), an organization whose mission was similar to my own. I'd searched the internet for Christian organizations that were involved with sports, and God led me to fca.org. As the nation's largest sports ministry, FCA has been reaching athletes and coaches for Christ since 1954 through camps, school "Huddles," ministry events, training, and resources. On their website, FCA offered the following statement:

> The Fellowship of Christian Athletes is touching millions of lives . . . one heart at a time. Since 1954, the Fellowship of Christian Athletes has been challenging coaches and athletes on the professional, college, high school, junior

high and youth levels to use the powerful medium of
athletics to impact the world for Jesus Christ. FCA is the
largest Christian sports organization in America. FCA
focuses on serving local communities by equipping,
empowering and encouraging people to make a difference
for Christ. ("Mission and Vision," fca.org)

I knew it was a perfect fit.

I sent an email through their contact page, and Jimmy Page was
the one who responded. Jimmy Page, one of FCA's vice presidents of
field ministry and the founder of their health and fitness ministry, lent
me his support and encouraged me that he would be behind me the
entire way. He and FCA joined the effort to help me tell my story and
touch those millions of lives. My relationship with Jimmy grew over
time, and I also became a contributing writer for FCA's "Daily Impact
Play" online devotionals, working with their magazine editor, Jill Ewert,
who was very encouraging and always offered me the platform to be an
inspiration to other believers.

———————————— ▣ ✦ ▣ ————————————

With all of the support flooding in, I felt empowered. More importantly, I felt the hand of God on me. If you've never experienced what
it's like to be used for something of eternal value, you're missing out.
Knowing you are making a difference in the world on behalf of the
Creator of the universe brings a fulfillment that can only be found by
saying yes to Him and doing whatever He asks. I felt like a mighty warrior in His army—like I was punching holes in the darkness, piercing
it with His light.

Because we are in a spiritual battle while here on earth, though, I
constantly had to fight the nagging voice of the antagonist. All of the
support was amazing, but with it came added pressure, and I started

to doubt whether I could handle the enormity of the MS Bodybuilding Challenge.

Inside, I asked myself if I had bitten off more than I could chew. Could I really compete in a bodybuilding contest while having MS and stand up against healthy bodybuilders? Could I even walk onto a stage and stand at all? How could I pose without losing my balance? Could I even build any real muscle while my body was destroying itself?

The questions, doubts, and uncertainty accumulated in my mind and sent me wandering down the path of negativity. The Goliaths were in front of me again. But thankfully, prayer was my weapon at hand.

So I prayed, and I prayed. I looked to Scripture for strength and to find affirmation that all things were possible with Christ. As I studied the Word, I could feel the Lord's presence in my heart and soul, and I knew there was a bigger purpose for my MS diagnosis.

It had been hard for me to realize that my life to that point hadn't been wasted or lost just because of the MS. Now I was beginning to see that the years I'd invested in serving God were not in vain. All of the good seeds that had been planted were meant to be harvested when He was ready. It was all in His timing, and the more I immersed myself in His Word, the more I accepted that truth. All of the inner strength I was finding was the result of taking hold of the hand of God. I prayed for confirmation that I could defeat this enemy; and with clarification only the Lord could give, I heard Him loudly tell me to . . . "Just do it!"

Chapter 6

TRAINING 101

The training program Darren had designed was grueling to say the least. Day after day, he pushed me to lift harder and be better. And, slowly but surely, I did. I had progressed enough in my training to where I had a good base going and was ready for more intensity. Now was the time to put a contest on the calendar and get started.

In order to avoid traveling, we looked at the lineup of contests being held near Orlando. I insisted on entering a National Physique Committee (NPC) show because, as the largest amateur bodybuilding organization in the United States, it would have the respect of the entire bodybuilding community and the highest level of competition.

Darren questioned my choice to take on an NPC show, as he knew, through his own victories and defeats, that the athletes who competed in these contests were huge, ripped, and full of performance-enhancing drugs. It was true that the sport had undergone a total transformation since the Schwarzenegger days of the seventies. The former well-proportioned, muscular physiques had been replaced by freakishly big, vascular, cut-up bodies.

When I competed in the eighties, Lee Haney won Mr. Olympia, but the unusually vascular and defined newcomer Rich Gaspari placed a very close second, paving the way for a new breed of competitor. Three decades later, veins were now standard and necessary in bodybuilders. Yesterday's pros were today's amateurs, and my chances of getting a trophy were obviously slim to none. Yet even with that knowledge, I wanted to make the point that no circumstance was too great and no giant too big to overcome. My goal to stand on an NPC stage was set, regardless of the odds.

After examining our options, we set our sights on the June 2009 NPC Mid-Florida Classic in Orlando, which was promoted by NPC Florida Central District Vice Chairman Deke Warner. The first thing Darren did after we made our decision was contact Deke to see whether he would lend his support. A competitive bodybuilder himself, Deke was all for it and even agreed to appear in a promo video we produced.

Deke was a great man who really wanted me to achieve my goal. He met with me on several occasions to discuss the show and how he felt I should handle the competition, and he continually told me that I would be a winner just by standing on the competition stage. He didn't want me to be concerned with what my competitors looked like. Instead, he told me that this was my challenge, not theirs, and that my victory was already taking place through my overall mission. Throughout the Challenge, Deke's words of encouragement would make an incredible difference in my mindset and help me to find peace whenever self-doubt crept in.

The support team was picking up momentum, and it fired me up. Darren and I were full steam ahead on the contest. Unfortunately, John's job forced him to train at different hours, but he continued to meet me for workouts whenever he could and encourage me as I stuck to Darren's routine. I told Darren not to baby me and to treat me like any other client getting ready to compete against other athletes. And, boy, did he listen! Darren's focus was on putting as much size on me as possible and pushing me to lift as much weight as I could, even though the MS was fighting against everything he was doing.

The training was brutal. I had little to no coordination, tremendous fatigue, and constant pain and numbness. It was extremely hard for me to grasp dumbbells and weight bars because I had very little grip, especially in my left hand. In order to complete the sets, I had to wrap straps around my wrists and then around the weights in order to keep them in place when my fingers gave, the hand fatigue set in, and I lost all feeling. In fact, on the last reps of the final sets, the weights would actually be held by the straps instead of my fingers.

There also was a troublesome stiffness in my left arm and hand that had remained since my attack in 2006. If you'd stuck a knife in my left arm, I wouldn't have felt it. While I could feel ninety percent of my right side, I could only feel twenty percent of my left. But even though I had little feeling on that side of my body when it came to touch, I still suffered pain from the pins-and-needles sensation.

While MS is a complicated disease to understand, the symptoms can be even more difficult to explain. How do you describe pain and numbness at the same time? It sounds contradictory if you've never experienced it, but it's simply being numb to the touch yet enduring painful tingling feelings inside your body.

In this condition, my left leg became the most problematic in training. Not only did it have the awful pins-and-needles sensation, it also faced extra effects from the disconnect in my brain. I would try my hardest to coordinate my left leg, but, no matter what I did, my leg would still drag. I just couldn't lift it the same way as my right leg. Performing leg movements during my workouts was like trying to sprint but only being able to walk.

Darren played a big role in my physically being able to complete the workouts. He would help me up from the leg press machine, coordinate my left side during squats and pull up on my left leg when it lagged in extensions or curls. During every workout—upper and lower body—both of my legs would shake, the left considerably more than the right. My whole body endured pain, pins and needles, shaking, and a weird internal vibration, and when I got overheated my skin would itch everywhere.

With so many symptoms, it's challenging just to stay sane when dealing with MS. And I'm not exaggerating. But I had to stay focused as best as I could. What choice did I have? The concentration and determination I put into the MS Bodybuilding Challenge helped me see the victory instead of the trial. I kept telling myself the truth that God had a purpose in it all, and I was at peace with that. It was His purpose; not mine. This was the way I needed to view the present moment, maintain hope for the future, and overcome the giant in my life.

On February 14, 2008, the game changed yet again. I was training without Darren and doing stiff-legged dead lifts after my quadriceps workout. About halfway through my second set, I felt my right hamstring start to burn. From years of bodybuilding experience, I knew this wasn't good. I was sure I had torn a muscle. Happy Valentine's Day!

Immediately, I dropped the bar and headed home to ice it. I didn't know how badly I had damaged the muscle, but I couldn't straighten my leg. All I could think was that the whole competition and Challenge was over. It scared the heck out of me to think that all of our hard work could be ended with just one injury.

Later that day I went to see Dr. Homan so that he could assess the damage. He was an incredible help and always found time to fit me in, even if it was after 5:00 p.m. and he was prepping to go home.

In his examination—thank God—he didn't see a major tear. He said that routine ice, stretching, massage, and rest would put me back on track. Just a few days after the injury I could tell it was getting better as my hamstring was sore but not painful. I worked around the injury and kept training upper body.

Through that scare, I learned a valuable lesson. Because I had MS, my weakened body was now more susceptible to injuries, and one serious one could flush the whole Challenge down the tube. So when I went back to the gym, I decided to be a lot smarter and not so much of a tough guy. My Superman days were over, and I had to face it. I needed to train hard but work smart and avoiding lifting more than my body could handle. That was the plan, anyway.

* * *

Within a short period of time my five foot ten inch body had gone from 165 pounds of deteriorated flesh to 195 pounds of muscle and bulk. The combination of training and nutritional supplements, protein powder and meals was working. Darren had impressed me as someone who followed through and knew how to accomplish his goals, and he was certainly doing his job with me. He was a martial arts champion as well as an amateur bodybuilding titleholder, and he had an inner drive as intense as mine. We were a great team.

At the end of February, Darren was ecstatic over the gains I had made and put a call into the local FOX network news anchor to tell her what I was doing. Instead of getting a return call from the anchor, we were surprised to get one from the head of programming, who called Darren and invited us to come on the morning news broadcast.

It was perfect timing. Because March is MS Awareness Month, we made the connection at just the right moment. Two weeks later, FOX 35 News in Orlando brought Darren and me in for an interview with anchor Lauren Laponzina. The few minutes we were given were just enough for us to tell our story, and it really helped validate our cause.

It wasn't long before emails and phone calls came flooding in. I was overwhelmed by the number of people who simply wanted to tell me I'd inspired them. Many of the contacts were from other MS patients, but I was also blessed to discover that our cause was touching the lives of those afflicted with other diseases and people in good health.

Around the same time Darren had reached out to FOX, he'd also emailed local radio host Bud Hedinger, who had a tremendous following in the central Florida area. Bud replied quickly to Darren, and on March 10, 2008, he interviewed me on his live radio show.

We spoke on air for more than ten minutes, and Bud was incredibly supportive of what we were doing. After the show, he posted my website on his blog, and once again the responses rushed in. It was all I could do to thank the Lord for what He was doing through me and through the battle against MS. Clearly there was a world full of hurting people out there who needed hope and inspiration, and He was using me to bring His light, love, and truth into those dark places.

⸻　　🔲　🔲　🔲　⸻

With all of the support and encouragement and the public spotlight that came with it, I knew I had to train like a madman. In order to reach the established goal, I would need to train as hard as I'd done in my twenties. While my body was vastly different, the intensity level needed to be every bit as high. Unfortunately, that was a big request for a body at war with MS.

If you ask any multiple sclerosis patient to name the single most constant symptom, they will say fatigue. We are always tired and weary, and we need more rest than a healthy person. Every day I struggled to get out of bed, and I had to really dig deep in order to make it into the gym. On many occasions, that battle proved to be more a test of my faith than a test of my strength.

Every time I trained, my symptoms would worsen and take hours to subside. With the nerve damage I'd sustained from the initial attack, it was obvious that regardless of how strong-willed I was, my symptoms were just not going to stop. No matter how hard my mind tried to convince me that I was still the young, healthy bodybuilder who could bend bars in the gym, my flesh said something else.

In order to keep moving forward in the journey, I had to totally recondition my thoughts to trust God for strength. Of course, I wanted miraculous healing, but I could see now that His plan was for me to overcome physical limitations. So when the disease would tell me one thing, I would have to tell it another based on His Word.

That mental battle was every bit as exhausting as the training. I had to daily, hourly choose to trust God and put my burdens on the shoulders of Christ. As a Christian, I found that the irresolution of the human mind and the struggles of the human flesh created some of my most intense battles. It was a constant wrestling match up there. On some days, I would be completely focused on the victory, and on others I would question my choice to take on the Challenge. Many times I wished that I had made my attempt quietly with no attention, and, when I started entertaining those thoughts, more fears would follow them regarding my ability to finish the goal. Then, if I let those thoughts take root, they would snowball into doubts surrounding my ability to train period, forgetting the competition all together.

It was war. The enemy was pounding my mind and assaulting me with lies, insecurities, and fear. He meant business, and it was clear that he didn't want to see this move forward, either for my sake or for those I was inspiring.

But it was in those dark times—in my weakest moments—that I felt the power of God's Word more than ever. I could have chosen to believe the voice of the deceiver, but I chose to allow the Lord to speak to me through Scripture.

The Bible contains so many words of encouragement and affirmations regarding the strength we have available in Him, and, when we fill our minds with these verses, we open a door for the Holy Spirit to empower us and help us overcome.

The Lord is my strength and my defense. (Exod. 15:2)

But David found strength in the Lord his God. (1 Sam. 30:6)

It is God who arms me with strength and keeps my way secure. (2 Sam. 22:33)

In His power, I learned that my weakness didn't have to create limitations. My body was His, and He could do whatever He wanted with it, regardless of pain or fatigue. It was Scripture that continued to strengthen me and propel me into the gym and through my workouts. And as a result, I grew stronger both physically and spiritually. My relationship with Christ deepened as I leaned on Him and allowed Him to fight for, beside, and through me.

Darren continued to train me four days a week, dividing up the muscle groups for the best results. In my competitive bodybuilding days I had been used to training six days a week for hours on end, but research had since shown that more time was needed between sessions in order to achieve maximum muscle growth and recovery. Based on the performances of today's competitors, it appeared that the studies were right.

For an old-school bodybuilder, that concept was difficult for me to believe. Darren wanted me use lighter weights, do more repetitions, complete slower movements, and take more days of rest, but I wanted to push heavy weights for fewer reps and use bursts of power. On the days when Darren wasn't with me, I snuck in my old training methods. Needless to say he wasn't happy with me and kept warning me that an MS-stricken fifty-year-old was more susceptible to injuries and that the last thing we needed was a torn muscle. He reminded me of my hamstring scare and how lucky I had been that it wasn't worse. "One injury could put an end to the MS Bodybuilding Challenge altogether," he'd say.

If only I'd listened.

——————————— ▧ ▧ ▧ ———————————

We were closing in on the one-year mark leading up to the June 2009 contest. Darren wasn't able to train me at the particular time I could get to the gym, so I was on my own for a chest and triceps workout one day.

I arrived at the gym and began warming up before my chest routine. I'd never been much for doing set after set of warm-ups and stretching before plunging in with the heavier weights. Instead, I would do one or two quick lightweight, high-rep movements, call it good, and get started. Call it being eager or impatient; either way, I wanted to get down to business.

The proper way to train, however, is to take enough time to warm up and stretch the muscles and to not start training while the muscles are still cold. This is where many of us old-school bodybuilders make a big mistake, and we've learned the hard way that getting blood into the muscles before an actual workout is essential to prevent injuries. We all think we're superhuman and can lift as much as we want, when we want, and we will never get hurt. Ironically, most of us have sustained tears and other injuries because of this pattern, yet we continue to avoid the warm ups. I don't know if that's being hard-headed or just plain stupid.

On this late spring day, I, as usual, did not warm up sufficiently. Instead, I laid down on the bench and started lifting with a first set of 225 pounds for twelve reps. I kept increasing the weight, moving to 275 for ten reps, 315 for eight, and then 365 for six. I should have stopped there as the last few reps of 365 were enough to end my bench press sets, but I was feeling very strong and decided to let my ego take over.

I hadn't lifted 400 pounds in more than twenty years; but on that day, I was going to relive my youth and show myself that even with MS I could out-lift the twenty-year-olds. I loaded the additional forty pounds to bring the total to 405. I positioned myself under the bar on the bench and adjusted my grip. Thankfully, I did have a spotter behind me in case I needed help, which was the smartest thing I did that day.

I lowered the weight onto my chest and lifted it for the first rep and then repeated it once more for the second. The bar went up, and I knew I had at least one more rep in me. I lowered the weight and pushed the bar upward. This rep was more of a struggle, but I did it. And now, because I had the security of a spotter, I thought I could even do one more.

I lowered the bar to my chest and started to press it up again. Right then, I heard a noise that sounded like someone tearing a piece of cloth. My right arm gave out, and the weight started to crash down on me while my left arm struggled to keep its end aloft. Before the right side of the bar hit my chest, my spotter grabbed it and heaved it back up onto the rack.

I sat up quickly and immediately knew I'd torn my right pectoralis (pec) muscle—not because of the pain, as I actually never felt it happening because of the numbness in my body, but because of the sound.

When I looked at my chest I saw blood starting to pool inside it and could see it already beginning to swell. I could barely move my right arm, and I knew this wasn't good.

As quickly as I could, I jumped into my car and grabbed the ice pack I had in my cooler. I always kept one handy for my protein drinks, so I applied it to the swollen area and headed straight to Dr. Homan's office. It was an intense twenty-minute drive, and all I could do was glance down and watch helplessly as the swelling increased and the internal bleeding worsened.

When I got to the doctor's office, the nurse took one look at my chest and rushed me into an exam room. Minutes later when Dr. Homan came in, he confirmed that the muscle was torn. However, due to the extreme swelling and internal bleeding, he couldn't determine how bad it was or rush to operate on it. He explained that the swelling and bleeding were normal with this type of injury and that it would stop eventually. The most he could do for now was bandage me up, give me pain pills and antibiotics and tell me to keep icing it and come back in a week.

I didn't want to know the answer, but I had to ask if this was the end of my training. Reluctantly, Dr. Homan told me that while it might not be the end, it was certainly going to result in a six-month recovery and a very slow return to training. It appeared that there was no way I would be able to compete in a year or maybe ever.

⬚   ⬚   ⬚

I left Dr. Homan's office with my head down in shame and anger. Why had I been such an idiot? I had risked everything to try to prove that I was as strong as I was in my twenties. My ridiculous pride had caused complete devastation.

When I got home, I sat on my couch with ice on my chest berating myself over and over for likely ending the MS Bodybuilding Challenge by being foolish. I was afraid to call Darren and tell him the news because I knew he'd say he'd told me so.

As the hours went by, the swelling increased and the bleeding continued to spread. It looked like my skin was going to burst open and explode with blood. I had no choice but to buck up and call Darren. Thankfully, as tough of a guy as he is, he also has a soft heart, and his response reflected that. Not once did he say that he'd told me it would happen. He was upset that all of our hard work wouldn't get us to the June 2009 contest, but he was more concerned about my health and how this would affect—or be affected by—my MS. He encouraged me that this was not the end and that once I healed we could set our sights on a contest further down the road.

Darren's positive attitude and support truly kept me from giving up completely that day, and I now had to put a lot of thought and prayer into our next move.

⬚   ⬚   ⬚

A week later, I went to my follow-up appointment with Dr. Homan. When he looked at the injury, he was visibly shocked. Starting at the midpoint of my right pec, I was black, blue, and red down my right side and my right arm. He said that the injury had been so severe and had bled so much that my body hadn't been able to absorb the blood fast enough. That's why it had spread as far as it had.

According to Dr. Homan, it was the worst tear he'd ever seen, and because it was still very swollen he couldn't tell how much of the pec was torn or if it was torn with or without the tendon. If the tendon had torn with the muscle, they could repair it by stretching the tendon back and reattaching it to the bone. However, if the tear was only in the muscle, the chances of repair were slight. Either way, Dr. Homan still predicted it would be six months before I'd even be able to attempt lifting light weights again.

Wanting to salvage whatever training base I could, I asked if lower body workouts and cardio training would be allowed. He gave me a cautious go-ahead but made me promise not to strain too hard and aggravate my injury. I gave him my word and made the decision to try lower body workouts the following week.

The next few weeks were torture as I went to the gym and had to refrain from training my upper body. Thankfully the swelling and discoloration were subsiding and, even though there was pain and stiffness, I could now move my right arm and chest. The one advantage of having MS was that the numbness helped me avoid much of the pain I would otherwise have felt.

As I wrestled with my mix of emotions and guilt, I continued to rely on God's Word as my cornerstone, battling daily to put the situation in His hands and trust Him. By focusing on Him and His truth, and through talking with Darren, I found the desire to get back on the horse and set a new contest goal. I still believed that there was a divine purpose in this and that this Challenge was the way God wanted to use me to inspire others. This was not the end.

Three weeks after the incident, I went back to Dr. Homan for another exam to find out when I could start training my upper body again. He examined the pec muscle and realized that it was indeed a muscle-only tear and not a tendon issue, meaning that if I trained too soon I would cause even more damage to the torn muscle, and then likely tear the tendon anyway. He asked me to get an MRI to assess the injury, which, based on my MRI history, was no easy chore, but was necessary in order to survey the damage. Once again I was pumped full of Valium and carted into the coffin.

When Dr. Homan reviewed the results, he was, with good reason, even more concerned than before. The test revealed that I had almost completely torn the pec off the bone. The muscle was ripped halfway into the center of my chest, leaving me with a balled-up half of a right chest. It was not a pretty sight, and Dr. Homan didn't think that any attempt to repair it would be successful. Instead, he wanted me to take the recovery slowly and start training lightly in about five months. After that point he would re-evaluate the possibility of operating.

This, of course, just did not cut it for me. I wanted to be back on the path of accomplishing my goal, and taking five months off wasn't in the game plan. So I did just what the doctor said not to do and headed back into the gym the next Monday morning.

The first workouts I did were extremely difficult and painful. I was stiff and could barely move my right side. In all of the upper body movements, I used light weights and worked around the tear. As the weeks went by, I pushed a little more and could eventually do chest exercises using the machines. Unfortunately, I now discovered that I'd damaged my left shoulder the day of the tear too, as it had been strained when trying to keep the bar from falling onto my chest.

In order to keep my left shoulder moving, Dr. Homan started painful cortisone injections. The needles he used were quite long and had to be inserted between the bone and the muscle. Even with my lack of overall feeling, the shots hurt and I dreaded them. More than anything, though, I dreaded the situation itself—it appeared as though everything was falling apart.

At this point, I was little more than a walking injury—a beat up man in an almost fifty-year-old body, who was battling MS. It was not the ideal situation for someone training to compete in a bodybuilding contest, but I was determined not to let anything stop me. Even if it killed me, I would continue training with a contest in sight and the MS Bodybuilding Challenge intact. If I could train through MS and a torn pec, I could certainly make it onto a bodybuilding stage—somehow, some way, some day.

Chapter 7

LOVE AT FIRST SITE

August and September are two of the hottest and most humid months in Central Florida, and we were right in the middle of them. The heat and humidity tremendously aggravated my disease, and the symptoms only got worse during workouts as my body temperature began to rise.

It started as tingling all over my body and eventually turned into itching. After that, it would escalate into a painful numbness everywhere. The workouts themselves had been challenging enough, but the climate just made it exasperating.

In those days of high temperatures, there was nothing I could do to avoid overheating. I would ice my body, take uncomfortably cold showers, and wear a cold bandana around my head while training. I prayed before every workout that I wouldn't feel these symptoms, but it was clear that endurance was how the Lord wanted to show His power instead.

In order to stay positive and remain focused on the goal and strong in my faith, I corresponded with many of the people who had been supporting me on the MS Bodybuilding Challenge website. I answered emails from other MS patients and continued to write devotionals for FCA. By staying focused on others, I could better see God's bigger plan in all of this—that it was about so much more than just my entering a bodybuilding contest. He was at work inspiring, challenging, and changing others through the testimony He was weaving in me.

In all of my prayers, I kept petitioning the Lord for peace in what was still a new life for me. It felt like it had been so long since I'd experienced deep rest in my soul, and I knew He wanted to offer that to me if only I would receive it. I prayed for a better understanding of His Word and His plan and focused on believing the truth of Scripture.

Over time this peace began to take root, and, as foreign as life had become to me over the past few years, I found that I was learning the ropes and adjusting to the new path. Soon, I started to reconsider the idea of companionship as well.

I was tired of fighting the battle alone as a single man. I wanted someone to share the journey with me, so I began praying for God to bring me a woman who would stand by me through it all—someone who could walk the journey with me and understand my drive to be the man He had called me to be. I needed a Christian woman who had an active relationship with the Lord and a passion for Him. I didn't want someone who just showed up to church on Sundays; I wanted a girl who genuinely lived her life for Christ.

In my first attempt at online dating, I'd jumped from one dating site to the next and given up in frustration, choosing, instead, to throw myself fully into training. I'd immersed myself in working out, eating, and resting and taken very little time out for dating or hanging out with friends. With my new outlook on life, though, I began asking the Lord to streamline the process and make it easier, perhaps sparing me the effort of having to go from site to site, sifting through women, trying to find the one Christian among them. That was just too draining.

That was when the Lord led me to the Christian dating site Christiansingles.com. I didn't even know Christian sites like that existed, but I knew that it would certainly increase my odds of finding someone who truly loved Christ. Plus, if it was the Lord who had sent me there, it had to be good.

Because I had no desire to travel in my quest for love, I decided that there was no sense in connecting with women who didn't live in the Orlando area. I limited my search criteria to include only those who were in range and began communicating with a few of the ones who surfaced. I talked to a couple of women, and, although they seemed nice, I didn't feel that God-breathed feeling that compelled me to pursue them.

One night, though, while searching through the list, I came across one who caught my eye. She was stunning! Immediately attracted to her, I clicked on her profile. The first thing I noticed was that she was from Southern California, and I wondered why she had popped up in my results even though she was outside of my selected location.

Without giving it a second thought, I clicked off of her profile and started to move on—until I heard the voice of God in my head tell me to go back to her picture. I know everyone hears the voice of God differently, but I clearly discerned Him telling me that she was the one.

"The one *what*, Lord?" I asked. "She doesn't even live in Florida!"

But I heeded the nudge and kept going back to "Kendra." I read her heartfelt bio over and over and knew in my heart that I needed to send her a message.

※ ※ ※

In my initial note, I told her that I liked what I read and that she seemed to have a relationship with Christ and a spirit for helping others. I gave her a short intro in which I shared my desire to be in the center of God's will and to do His work, and then I waited for a reply.

When I received it, I was shocked. Among other things that were positive in nature, she had written to "quit the email." What? How could she tell me to stop emailing her when I had poured out my heart and expressed my love for God? I wasn't about to sit idly by on that one, especially not when God had told me she was the one. So my reply was simple: "Did I scare you away?"

I wondered whether the profile picture I'd been using, which featured me sitting on a custom chopper with my tattoos showing, communicated to her that she needed to stay as far away from me as possible. Or maybe my Florida address had been a deterrent. Either way, I had to find out.

Much to my delight, she responded with a humorous story. Apparently, she'd been typing quickly when she'd responded and had written "quit" instead of "quite." According to Kendra, she had a tendency to type quickly and send out emails without proofreading them or using the spell checker. We both laughed about it and immediately began sending messages back and forth getting to know each other as best we could over the internet.

I soon found out that Kendra had also made an internal commitment not to communicate with those outside her local area, but that didn't stop us now. Our connection was too good to pass up.

I will say that Kendra was cautious and presented a bit of a challenge—at least for a few days. It took some convincing to get her to give me her phone number, but when she did, we couldn't stop talking. We felt connected immediately, and after our initial phone conversation, which lasted five hours, we both hung up with smiles on our faces. According to Kendra, she said to herself right then, "I think I just met my husband."

It was important to me that I be up front and honest with Kendra from the start. I let her know I'd been diagnosed with MS and that I was choosing to fight the disease through bodybuilding. I told her boldly that I would never be in a wheelchair, even though I couldn't guarantee the truth of that statement.

"Coincidently," Kendra turned out to be a home health nurse who had experience with MS patients. She knew all about its devastating effects, and yet she still chose to date me. Clearly, she was an incredible woman. She knew MS was a progressive disease and that, if we stayed together, it could not only send me to that dreaded wheelchair but also require her to push it.

Knowing she was an exceptional woman, I wasted no time in making plans to fly to California to meet her. It was important that Kendra's three grown children, Kara, Christian, and Kalie, have the opportunity to meet me. I was sure they thought their mom was crazy for getting involved with a stranger from Florida, and to be honest it did sound a little nuts. But this was where our faith in God made all the difference. We chose to walk by faith and trust Him instead of looking at the perceived logic of the situation. If it was His will that we be together, we wanted to know.

That first trip eventually led to more, and, after seven months of going back and forth, we both knew that there was no one else in the world for us. On April 4, 2009, I made my last trip out to California, bringing along my children to witness our wedding.

The next day Kendra and her dog, Kammie, moved back to Florida with us. Kendra and I both knew our plans would be to eventually return to Southern California where we could build my entertainment business, but, for now, her bonding with my children was more important. She wanted to cultivate relationships with them as their new stepmom, and it was a great blessing to me that she wanted to be involved in their lives. Clearly, God had blessed me with the one—*His* one.

So began our life's journey together. And now, along with all of the "normal" aspects of being newly married, Kendra found herself right in the middle of the MS Bodybuilding Challenge and all it entailed—a role that she embraced with support, encouragement, understanding, and love.

I had asked the Lord to bring me a partner in life, and instead He delivered me a woman with the heart of an angel.

Chapter 8

THE FIRST CONTEST

After our wedding, Kendra and I settled into our home a few miles down the road from where my children lived with their mother. Shortly thereafter, we went on a honeymoon to Costa Rica where we had the chance to relax and enjoy some time alone before Kendra started her new job as a home health nurse, and I got back to work on *Hog Heaven*, and, of course, back to training.

Because of the high temperature and humidity in Costa Rica, my MS symptoms flared, and I struggled each day to coordinate movements and fight fatigue. Certainly, it wasn't a typical honeymoon, but Kendra, with her nurturing soul, made the trip so much less stressful. By the time we left I had a deeper appreciation for the amazing wife God had given me.

As soon as we returned to Florida, I called Darren and told him I was ready to put a new contest on the calendar. Since Deke Warner had been supporting my cause, we wanted to pick an NPC show he was promoting. The contest that appeared to fit the schedule best was the Florida State Bodybuilding Championship on August 22, which I figured was just enough time for me to diet and prepare. Darren adjusted my training routine and diet to gear up for the competition, and the countdown began.

─────────────── ▣ ▣ ▣ ───────────────

Back in the gym I pushed hard trying to maintain as much muscle mass as I could while also dropping body fat. Dieting while training is hard enough for a healthy, seasoned bodybuilder, but for a fifty-year-old guy with MS who hadn't trained for competition in more than twenty years, it was arduous.

My diet consisted of six meals a day and centered mostly on protein, vegetables, and supplements. I ate four solid meals of fish, lean red meat, or white-meat turkey or chicken, including a small amount of carbs at the first two. Carb servings were usually a cup of brown rice, a sweet potato, or Ezekiel 4:9 Sprouted Grain Bread. My vegetables were mainly broccoli, spinach, or other leafy greens, and I consumed handfuls of pills containing omega-3 fatty acids, vitamins, minerals, and CLAs (conjugated linoleic acids), which would help burn fat. Finally, I would have two protein drinks between meals—Myofusion by Gaspari Nutrition—to round out the day's nutritional needs.

My calorie total hovered around two thousand per day, which was ridiculously low for me, and my fats came only from a teaspoon of olive oil here or there. With such a low-calorie, low-carb, low-fat diet, I lacked energy for anything other than workouts. Darren implemented a cardio routine to help burn fat, but with such low-carb intake and the basic fatigue of MS, I was too exhausted to do cardio either before or after weights. Plus, cardio was just embarrassing for me, stumbling along on the treadmill or battling an interrupted stride on the elliptical machine. In lieu of cardio, I increased the intensity and pace of my regular workouts to help speed up my metabolism. If I was going to burn fat, it would have to be with weights and diet alone.

━━━━━━━━━━ ▨ ▨ ▨ ━━━━━━━━━━

Like most men, I love eating—and eating a lot of food at once. It's hard to keep me away from ice cream and carbs, but at this point I had no choice. I dug in and focused on the fact that I only had a few months to drop my waist size.

The calorie total was a major adjustment. I'd been used to eating five thousand calories every day, so dropping to two thousand felt like starving. I looked like a rabbit, constantly trying to get full by eating vegetables.

At first, my body craved carbs and that delicious chocolate, chocolate chip ice cream at Cold Stone. But, once I set my mind to it, I stayed focused. I would not be broken by food. When Kendra and I would go out to a restaurant, I always asked that my meal be prepared without salt and made as bland and low-fat as possible. As a fan of carbs herself, Kendra would enjoy pasta or rice while I chewed on carrot sticks, and she often looked at me and said she couldn't believe my level of discipline. Every time I watched her enjoy that warm bread and butter, I thought the same thing.

━━━━━━━━━━ ▨ ▨ ▨ ━━━━━━━━━━

On May 21, 2009, Bud Hedinger invited me back to his live radio show to discuss how the training was going and find out what had happened to the original contest date. It was a great chance for me to talk about the pec injury and how it had challenged me to push through adversity. It also gave me an opportunity to discuss the new competition date and how our revised plans were progressing, letting others know that I was still set on completing the mission.

As in my first interview with Bud, he was supportive and sincerely amazed at what I was accomplishing in spite of multiple sclerosis. And, just like before, the emails and phone calls streamed in and showered me with encouragement. No one wanted me to give up. God was using my journey to encourage many people with and without MS, and I didn't want to let them down.

Again, shortly after the interview, I began to experience overwhelming levels of doubt. It was becoming a vicious cycle whenever I seemed to be gaining confidence. The enemy would work overtime in my mind to make me question what I was doing and why I was pushing my body to such extremes. They say that the mind is the devil's playground, and he was certainly having a good ol' time in mine.

Once again I prayed in desperation for the Lord to give me the strength, stamina, and determination to finish the quest. It felt like each stage of the journey was harder than the one before, and I was certainly in a rough spot. The training fires had been turned up regarding diet and weights, my MS symptoms were constant, especially regarding fatigue, and the pressure of the pending contest was bearing down.

In a moment of sincere questioning, I looked at Kendra and asked her opinion regarding whether I should keep going. Her response made it so clear why the Lord had chosen her for me. Many women would have told me to quit, but Kendra spoke words of faith. She told me to look into my heart and ask myself if I still believed that this was God's will for me. If it was, then I should continue to do what needed to be done. She would stand behind me either way. Then she threw in one more bit of truth, saying that if God had started me on this path, He had a plan for me to finish it.

Kendra says that one of the main reasons she married me was because she had never seen anyone with as much determination. I love hearing that. Determination is a quality I value in myself, and it's one that comes from the belief that if I'm given a goal I need to do whatever it takes to achieve it. As a Christian, all of the glory is God's, anyway. I'm just a vessel for Him to use when making His point.

——————————— ▨ ▨ ▨ ———————————

It was now the end of May, and we were approaching the three-month mark leading up to the show. On one particular day, I went to the gym for another grueling leg workout that would push my body, mind, and soul. Legs were the most difficult body part for me to train, not only because of the stamina required, but also because of my lack of coordination and the painful numbness on my left side.

I finished one set of leg presses with ten forty-five-pound plates loaded on each side of the press machine and grabbed the sides of the machine to steady myself. I slowly got up, basically crawling out from under the apparatus. The total I'd been pushing, including the weight of the press slide, had been more than one thousand pounds. When I finally made it to a standing position my legs started shaking furiously. It wasn't the normal kind of shake that comes with a hard workout; it was the kind of shake that stemmed from MS-stricken nerves.

As I stood there trying to coordinate my legs, I looked around the gym at the other bodybuilders. They were all healthy. They stood strong and steady on their legs. They didn't have to hold onto the machines to keep from losing their balance.

In that moment, it hit me like never before that I was disabled. My stomach started to sink as if it was full of lead, and I felt hopelessness begin to creep up upon me. A barrage of doubts assaulted my mind, and

I literally had to stop and answer the question, *Is this really me? Is this who I am now? Will the real David Lyons please stand up?*

Yes, it was me. I was the one who couldn't feel my left leg or foot other than the tingling and pain. Even though the mirrors showed that I was standing, it felt as if my leg was dangling in midair. I shook my head in frustration, baffled by the moment and the sudden wave of emotions. I did my best to coordinate the movement in my extremities and carry on, but I could feel a depression trying to take me over, so I stopped right there and began to acknowledge God. Would I look at my circumstances or look to Him? I resolved, *I choose to look at the Lord!* My faith in God and the victory He was bringing was bigger than what I was facing, both at that gym and in my life.

I went home after that workout and evaluated what I'd experienced. I realized that the time during those intense moments was when I really needed to search my heart and find my faith—faith that went beyond understanding—faith that would tell me there was a reason for what I was going through and that God would deliver me if I trusted Him. While I might not be able to see where He was taking me at the time, I could still know that it was going to be good. That day, even if I couldn't feel the floor beneath me, I could still choose to believe that my path was a blessed one because it was orchestrated by the Lord of lords and King of kings.

I opened my Bible to 1 Kings 2:4: "And that the LORD may keep his promise to me: 'If your descendants watch how they live, and if they walk faithfully before me with all their heart and soul, you will never fail to have a man on the throne of Israel.'" While I wasn't preparing descendants for a seat on the throne of Israel, I was walking faithfully, despite my circumstances. Based on His Word, I believed that faithfulness would assure me of God's victory, whatever that meant.

It had been an incredibly challenging day. There were several of those along the way, and they always made me want to scream, "Why me, Lord?!" That day, I really wondered how I could continue to live life with a disease-filled body. I truly thought I'd reached the end of my rope. But in God's Kingdom, I found that there was no end to the rope. He always had more to spare and would cast me a line whenever I needed it. My only job was to grab on.

As the competition drew closer, my torn pec continued to complicate things. I had to constantly work around the injury in order to keep from tearing the muscle even more or damaging the tendon, which, at this point, was the only thing connecting my shoulder to my chest. The scar tissue that had formed in the area also wasn't as pliable as muscle, which made it difficult to move. Plain and simple, my right pec was a mess, and it was affecting almost all of my upper body exercises. Each movement had to be altered in some way in order to avoid aggravating the pec. I couldn't pull my arms back too far or stretch the muscle too much, and I certainly couldn't push too much weight.

There was no way around it. At contest time, that part of my body was not going to match the rest, and I was going to look strange. I kept thinking to myself that now I would be entering a bodybuilding contest with MS *and* a deformity. This was insane!

Plus, let's be honest here. Even if I was a healthy bodybuilder, I would have needed a lot more time to train and prepare for a contest than I was giving myself, especially when I hadn't stepped on stage in more than twenty-five years and was coming back from a severe injury. I simply had to come to grips with the fact that I wouldn't look like I wanted to on stage. If I could just put that feeling of inadequacy aside, I would be fine.

But my ego was a monster, and I was having a really hard time bringing it down.

I had to keep reminding myself of the basic fact: I had a disease that made muscle regeneration difficult, and no amount of training or dieting would change that. I needed to keep everything in perspective and stay fixed on my true goal, which was to show the world the power of God in the face of human limitation. They needed to know that being diagnosed with MS was not a death sentence; it was a chance to embrace His strength and power to overcome.

That was the mission. It wasn't about how great I looked, but about how great God was.

After a month of strict low-calorie dieting, fast-paced training, and higher reps, I still found it hard to drop the fat that had accumulated around my stomach during all my years of not watching what I ate. Since I still wasn't doing any cardio, Kendra suggested we put a treadmill in the house and that I slowly start incorporating it into my routine in an environment where I felt comfortable finding my coordination. This way, even if I stumbled, no one would see me and I could push myself as hard or as little as I wanted without my ego getting in the way.

The home treadmill turned out to be a great idea. Every night, long after I'd worked out at the gym and had recouped my energy, I would get on the treadmill for thirty minutes. At first, all I could manage was a slow-paced walk with my left leg dragging; but it wasn't long before I was able to get my legs to stay in pace and maintain a moderate run.

It wasn't easy, of course, and cardio proved to be a beastly endeavor when it came to MS. I got overheated quickly, and I would often lose my balance. In fact, there were times when I lost my coordination entirely and almost fell off the machine. At the end of every session I would need hours to recuperate while waiting for the pins and needles to stop coursing through my body. And there would also be a strange vibrating feeling radiating inside me, which took a very long time to dissipate. But cardio training was something I had to do if I was going to get into condition for the contest. I did what I could to mentally block out what my body was experiencing and put it in God's hands.

At the end of June, with only two months to go before the Florida State Bodybuilding Championship, I had dropped another ten pounds. I could now see the kind of definition in my muscles that I hadn't seen in years. It was incredible progress, but I still had plenty of fat to burn and not much time. Because of the calorie reduction, I had lost some muscle size and was hovering around 190 pounds, which was down from my beginning weight of 216. I was still at a reasonable size for my height, but I knew I had to step up the cardio and burn more fat.

What was really bothering me, though, was the look of my torn pec. The more fat I lost, the more I could see the deformity of the tear, and it made me nervous. I didn't want to get on stage with an awkward-looking chest. In my previous bodybuilding days, that had been my best feature. Now, half of my right side was torn in toward the middle of my chest muscle, and it only became more apparent as I dropped more fat.

By the end of July, I could see even more drastic changes in my physique. Some were fantastic, like my abs being tighter in my thirty-two-inch waist; and some, like the loss of my overall muscle size, were not so great. I could tell my muscles were shrinking as my weight dropped below 180 pounds. This made me wonder whether I was becoming too small for competition, especially since I knew I still needed to lose more fat in order to achieve the desired level of definition.

With that becoming an increasing issue in my mind, I called Darren and asked him for advice. He asked me to come in and meet with him and his friend Jim Schreiber. Jim and his wife, Tina, had been competing for years and both were champions at the amateur level.

Because of our conflicting schedules, Darren and I hadn't seen each other in a while. And when he and Jim saw me, they both had the same response. I had dropped a lot of body fat in a short amount of time, which had resulted in the loss of some quality muscle mass. What we all knew was that bodybuilding—especially contest-prep bodybuilding—was a science. It takes a person years to know how his or her body will respond to specific training routines and diets, and, because this contest was my first in this condition, I was an experiment.

When we started, we had no idea what would be the best way to train a body battling MS, and my muscle tear and recovery had only complicated matters. Now it appeared that the timeframe for an August competition had been too ambitious a goal. It was just too taxing on my body. But there was no way I was stopping now. We had one month to go, and I was going to finish the challenge.

I told Darren and Jim that I'd keep moving forward, and, thankfully, they both supported my decision. They reminded me that this contest wasn't about my looking like I did in my twenties or about being the biggest and best bodybuilder on stage. It was about doing what most people said couldn't be done and becoming the only fifty-year-old bodybuilder with MS to ever compete in an NPC contest.

Even with their encouragement, I was still really worried about my size. The reflection in the mirror revealed that I was only a fraction of what I'd been when we'd started. Jim could tell I was losing steam and immediately offered to meet me at Darren's gym early in the morning and help me train. Jim was a great guy, and he committed to doing whatever he could to help me get to the stage on August 22.

⊡   ⊡   ⊡

The next day, Jim showed up at the gym with a new workout drink for me in hand. And from that day on, Jim never missed a workout with me—or a workout drink. Darren would also sneak over while he was working and help us through the routines.

Just as crunch time was rolling in, God increased my support team again. There was no way we were giving up now. I had Kendra at home cooking my meals, making sure I did my cardio, and cheering me on the whole way. Darren and Jim were pushing me through the workouts and calling me every day to encourage me and check in on my condition and training. Those guys were doing everything they could to keep as much muscle on me as possible while helping me drop the last of the fat. By the time we approached the contest, there were veins coming through my skin over my abs, which meant my body fat had decreased significantly.

⊡   ⊡   ⊡

Even with the progress, I still battled my intense ego. As a Christian, I believe there is no room for ego in God's Kingdom, and pride is certainly the downfall of many. I struggle in this area in many respects; and as the contest day quickly drew near, I worried about embarrassing myself by standing against seasoned, healthy competitors, especially at a high level of competition.

In an effort to find some affirmation, I called Deke Warner to talk, and he said he'd be happy to meet me for dinner that week.

Deke hadn't seen me since we'd filmed the MS Bodybuilding Challenge promo at the beginning of the journey, and he was impressed at how far I'd come. As we dined—me with a plate full of bland chicken breast and broccoli—I expressed my hesitation about the contest and my fears about standing up against these men. Because Deke is a no-nonsense kind of guy, he looked me straight in the eye and asked, "Dave, why are you doing this? Are you doing this to beat bodybuilders who compete year after year, or are you doing this to beat MS?"

While I knew the answer immediately, I still wrestled with it. My ego told me that I needed to beat those guys, but my soul told me the truth. Obviously I wasn't going to win the contest—not even close. I would be blessed just to be up there competing against all odds—defying what logic said was impossible.

Yes, the answer was that I was competing to make a point, not to win a contest, but there was still—and maybe always would be—an inner desire to be the best. It was just something I would have to put in the Lord's hands every day. Mentally and emotionally I didn't want to be in my own reality as a fifty-year-old man with an incurable disease, and it was hard to come to terms with the facts; but Deke reminded me that there was also success to be found simply in breaking new ground. No one had ever done what I was doing at an NPC level-five contest. Never had a man with MS at age fifty walked onto a stage and flexed with the best bodybuilders in the organization. On behalf of all MS patients and disease victims, I would be achieving a victory that had nothing to do with trophies or titles.

We finished dinner, and Deke reiterated his support of my cause, making sure I knew and understood that he was proud of what I was doing. I don't think Deke was aware of this at the time, and he may not know it now, but his dinner and his reinforcement of the goal made all the difference in my staying the course.

The final two weeks of training and dieting were fourteen of the longest, most difficult days of my life. I had been at it for so long and had taxed my nervous system and muscles to such a degree that they seemed to have reached their breaking point. Facing MS head-on while preparing for a bodybuilding contest was not for the faint of heart. Thankfully, Christ's power inside me set me apart from that crowd. Even though the stress and fatigue were like nothing I had ever experienced and I was drained in every way imaginable, I knew He would carry me through to the contest.

MS had put so many limits on my body, mind, and spirit that, without the unlimited power of God and fervent, consistent prayer, I never could have endured to the contest day. At times, I was in so much pain and so exhausted that I wouldn't even tell Kendra what I was feeling. I didn't want her to worry any more than she already was. Just watching me going through it all and doing her best to encourage and support me was hard enough on her. I thought that if she actually knew how I was feeling she might crack.

During every workout over that last month of training, my entire left side rebelled against me. My left leg shook so badly that doing any standing movements was more demanding than ever. I would have to readjust my stance midway through every set or else the shaking would get out of control. And holding a dumbbell or barbell with my left hand was every bit as challenging as the workout itself. Many times, I would run out of steam at the end of a set and have to drop the weight due to the lack of grip on that side. It was incredibly frustrating, which just made me even more determined to train through it.

After upper-body workouts, I would leave the gym with no ability to hold onto anything and in the kind of pain that I wouldn't wish on my worst enemy. On the days I worked legs, I had to crawl and hobble out of the equipment and limp my way out of the gym dragging my left leg.

So many times, I almost fell over because of my lack of coordination. I was, without a doubt, challenging my MS-stricken body beyond its ability. I wasn't giving it any time to deal with the nerve damage it had sustained, and it was crying out for rest. I cursed the disease every time I trained, demanding things from my body that it just didn't want to deliver anymore. Once again, I was fighting for my sanity.

I refused to let Jim take it easy on me as my trainer during those final, grueling weeks. I knew it was tough on him to watch me suffer and drive myself as hard as I did, but I told him that no matter what it looked like, he mustn't worry; just let me train through the pain.

Jim proved to be a great trainer and friend. From the moment we started training together, he took me through every rep and every set up to the very end. Darren, who was also training for the over-forty division of the contest, stayed by my side as well and jumped in on our workouts as often as possible. He and I were both losing a lot of body fat and getting pretty cut up.

Shedding all of the fat, though, seemed to confuse my body, and it felt like it just didn't know quite how to respond. Obviously, I needed a certain amount of fat to live, so with my quest to shed so much of it, my body battled back to try and retain as much of it as it could. And with so many years between serious training periods and my battle with MS, my body had basically gone into survival mode.

In the absence of fat, my body was using its muscle tissue for additional energy, and I was down to around 170 pounds. I looked "flat," as they say in bodybuilding, and I knew I wasn't as big as I needed to be for the contest. My muscles looked small and not as pumped up as they should have been. The only solution we had was to start carb-loading, which would bring fullness to the muscles.

No matter what we did, though, I knew I'd still be too small to seriously compete against the monsters that would be on that stage. Every time I looked in the mirror I fought that mental and spiritual battle. With every gaze, I'd wish the man staring back at me had the nineteen-inch arms and fifty-two-inch chest that I'd had in the eighties. Between my longing to be the powerful man I'd once been and my moments of acceptance regarding the present, I lived in a constant state of flux between compliance and rejection—defeat and victory. At times it was torture. I felt like I was going crazy, and, as the contest drew closer, depression became a constant threat.

Those closest to me could see what was going on, and they responded with amazing support. Darren and Jim held me up physically and mentally and encouraged me to keep going, while Kendra—well—Kendra was my rock. Whenever I lagged, she sensed it and helped me find my strength in Christ and lean on Him again. It was a message I needed to hear often, because in my human strength this was not possible either physically or mentally. If left to myself, I would have given up, given in, or given myself over to depression, but I wasn't alone. I had God's power inside me, His people beside me, and His Word to fuel me, enabling me to "stand on the heights" (2 Sam. 22:34).

As the contest date closed in, the battle raged on, but I knew the Lord was not to be stopped. I could feel Him telling me that this test was one of perseverance and faith, and if I stayed the course, it would prove that, through Him, all things are possible.

———————— ✦ ✦ ✦ ————————

On contest day, Darren and I had to get up early and drive to Dr. Phillips High School in Orlando, which was where we would be competing. Prejudging started at 10:00 a.m., and the contest would start at 6:00 p.m. We were in for a long day.

During pre-judging, the contest judges would take their first looks at the contestants before the evening's final so that they could be familiar with our bodies before we went through our poses that night. Darren and I arrived at 9:00 a.m. and went backstage to pump up and put on our posing oil. Jim and Tina were already there waiting to help us get ready.

When I got backstage, I was absolutely flooded with memories. It seemed like a hundred years since the last time I'd been backstage for a bodybuilding contest, either to compete myself or to assist someone else. And while it hadn't been a full century, it had been since 1983 when I'd helped my friend Steve Adell get ready for the NPC Junior National Bodybuilding Championship.

※　※　※

The 1980s had been a decade of the change in the bodybuilding world—one that ushered in a new breed of bigger, more defined competitors who had incredible vascularity. And, ever since then, it has just gotten more and more competitive. Steve was a big guy with great symmetry who had been compared to Arnold Schwarzenegger, but on that day he had taken the stage against a young man who was so muscularly dense and so vascular that he could not be matched. His name was Rich Gaspari, and he not only won the contest that day, he also set a new bar in bodybuilding competition. A year later, Gaspari turned pro and, at age twenty-one, became the youngest man ever to win the Mr. Universe contest. He would go on to place second three times in the Mr. Olympia contest—the world's ultimate professional bodybuilding competition—and compete until the late nineties, before being inducted into the IFBB Hall of Fame in 2004.

As a bodybuilder, I paid attention to the changes in the sport. Because I had been so closely tied to Steve in 1983 when Rich Gaspari started his ascent, Rich's career had always inspired me. Just like any other sport, bodybuilding comes with its own unique culture, and those who compete in it have a certain set of heroes and icons who have broken barriers and achieved great things. In my opinion, Rich was one of those guys. After his successful career, Rich went on to establish Gaspari Nutrition, one of the largest and most successful bodybuilding supplement companies in the industry. He and his wife, Liz, were wonderful people, and they had sponsored me during my preparation for the MS Bodybuilding Challenge by providing cutting-edge, pre-contest supplements.

It was a huge blessing to receive such support and encouragement from others in the sport, including a man I'd admired and respected for two and a half decades. But as I looked around, I realized that at 170 pounds, I was still an infant compared to the 230-pounders in the room. The sport had changed so much, and I wasn't in its range.

In the eighties, a contest-shape bodybuilder was considered big if he weighed more than 200 pounds. In fact, Arnold was around 220 when he was Mr. Olympia. Now, I was in a contest full of amateurs who would have been considered professionals in my day. These guys were huge, cut, and vascular. I think the smallest competitor in my age division was right at 200 pounds. What was I doing here?

* * *

All of the memories involving Rich and the evolution of bodybuilding came rushing back as I stood backstage preparing. Honestly, I was so flooded by the past that it was hard to concentrate on what I was doing. The sights, the sounds, the smells—all were new but still the same. I couldn't believe how so many of the same emotions had stayed with me over the years. If only my eighties body had done the same.

As Tina helped me get ready and I stood there daydreaming, a tall competitor in his fifties came up to me and asked, "Are you David

Lyons?" When I told him I was, he hugged me and introduced himself as Mike Ives. He told me he'd seen my MS video on YouTube and thought what I was doing was incredibly inspiring. In fact, Mike was so excited to meet me that he started bringing other competitors over and introducing them to me. Everyone was encouraging and seemed to be genuinely moved by my story. They were supportive and humble, and it truly touched my heart.

To be honest, this outpouring shocked me. My memories of bodybuilding competition were of extreme rivalry between the athletes who viewed each contest as a war. I even remembered guys messing with each others' posing oil in order to get an edge on their competitors. But on that day there was a spirit of camaraderie, not battle.

As I talked with Mike, I learned that he had been competing for awhile and had gone from a very skinny, out-of-shape man to a ripped, competitive amateur bodybuilder. He had such a great spirit about him, and I could tell from the start that he was a Christian. We bonded quickly and our conversation soon turned toward Christ and how He had changed both our lives and given us the strength to overcome life's obstacles. Mike encouraged me so much that I knew instantly he was a gift from God.

It was a miracle that a man like Mike had been sent to the same contest, placed in the same area, and found me in the very moment when my memories and fears were threatening to overtake me. God knew I was in desperate need of spiritual encouragement, and our encounter helped me get past the nervousness and anxiety I experienced as I looked around at the monsters in my division. Once again, the Lord had rescued me and renewed my Kingdom vision.

We waited for what felt like an eternity as each class was called on stage to do the mandatory poses for the judges. When my class, which was the over-thirty division, was called, we lined up in the order of our given number. At number seventy, I was in the middle of the line, sandwiched between two animals who looked like they'd never missed a workout or a meal. Deke had allowed me to compete in the over-thirty division as a way of showing that I could compete with anyone, and we were certainly aiming high.

I wasn't tremendously confident to begin with, but now, on stage, I was experiencing massive doubt. It was as if I'd forgotten all about the encouragement of the morning. Each MS symptom seemed to be heightened by my stress, and, as I stood in line, my left leg shook and my extremities tightened.

Now before the judges, we were to go through the poses they asked for and then walk off the stage. I stood there on the hardwood floor in the auditorium and listened to them call out the poses from their seats behind a long table. I was so focused on not losing my balance and on hearing the correct poses that I never even bothered to count the number of judges. I think there were six.

One of them was a familiar face. Peter Potter, who was the NPC Florida vice chairman at the time, had been a part of the organization for many years, and I'd known him since the late eighties when I helped a friend train at Peter's gym, the Hollywood Health Club. In 1992 I purchased that gym from Peter, and now, seventeen years later, I was standing on a bodybuilding stage putting myself under his judgment. I have no idea whether he remembered me, but knowing he was on the panel only fueled my thoughts of the past and made me realize how much had changed.

The morning's crowd consisted mainly of family members and close friends. The full crowd of spectators, avid bodybuilders, and fans would

show up for the finals that evening. There was no music, bright spotlight, or hoopla for this part of the show; it was just the competitors out
on the cold floor, vulnerable to the judges' opinions.

This part of the day was all business, and most of the decisions
regarding who placed and in what order were determined by the morning's pre-judging. Anyone could pretty much tell who the top three athletes were right there, but the individual posing routines that night would
determine where they fell in the final placement. Unlike the others, I
wasn't concerned with placing. I couldn't be. If I let myself go there mentally, I would be crushed. I had to keep reminding myself that my place
was that I was there at all—competing—standing next to healthy guys
twenty years my junior and making a stand in my battle against Goliath.

I was on stage for ten minutes, but it felt like ten days. Overall, it took a
couple of hours for all 150-plus competitors to get through the process.
As it turned out, that year's show was the biggest in the history of the
competition. I'd just had to pick the largest and highest level of show to
be in. Even the pre-judging crowd of friends and family was larger than
normal because of the large number of competitors. It was intimidating
to say the least, and all I could do was stand there with my thoughts as I
waited for Darren to go through his mandatory poses for the over-forty
class. When he was done, we went home to rest and get ready for the
evening's finals.

On the drive home, we talked about how we thought we looked, how
massive the competitors were, and how many guys were in the lineup.
Darren wasn't feeling very confident in his performance and his condition that year, so he was apprehensive. In 2007, he'd won the contest's

over-thirty-five class, and he had been hoping to do well in 2009. After seeing the competition, though, he wasn't so sure he'd place.

Obviously, I knew I was being blown away by the other guys in my class and that the contest was simply out of my league. I'd known that all along. But now, actually seeing it was creating a wave of doubt that I'd accomplished anything at all. What was the point? If I couldn't be a serious contender, why was I even doing this? Did anyone care whether I was up there if I couldn't make a legitimate run at it? Was all of that talk about true victory just nonsense? By the time I walked into the house and saw Kendra standing there anxiously awaiting an update, I felt completely defeated.

I knew that my faith and confidence should be coming from Christ and that my ego needed to be checked at the curb. God had never promised an easy road, and He never once told me that my faith wouldn't be tested. In fact, His Word said just the opposite—that I would experience great challenges—but that He would see me through them all.

> Consider it a great joy, my brothers, whenever you experience various trials, knowing that the testing of your faith produces endurance. But endurance must do its complete work, so that you may be mature and complete, lacking nothing. (James 1:2–4 HCSB)

> Today you are going into battle against your enemies. Do not be fainthearted or afraid; do not be terrified or give way to panic before them. For the LORD your God is the one who goes with you to fight for you against your enemies to give you victory. (Deut. 20:3–4)

I wanted so badly to believe those words, but, as everyone who walks a journey with God knows, fear and doubt are relentless enemies. At that moment, they were stampeding my willpower and shooting arrows through my heart. I couldn't do it.

"How'd it go?" Kendra asked. I'm sure my face said it all before I even uttered one word. There I was, standing in my living room, looking at Kendra and telling her that I felt this contest was bigger than my ambition. The Goliath was too big, and I was one David who didn't have the confidence to defeat him.

My words were incoherent, and I was talking complete nonsense. Finally, in my fatigue from the morning, exhaustion from the disease, and weakness from lack of nutrition, I said the unthinkable: "Kendra, I don't want to go back on that stage tonight." I told her I was too small and that I didn't have the conditioning to match these monsters who had been training consistently for the past twenty years. I was like a novice compared to them—a novice with only half a right pec to flex. "Let me just eat a pizza and call it a day. I tried."

Kendra's sweet demeanor quickly switched gears. It was time for hard truth. "You are not a quitter, Dave," she said. "Since the day I met you, I have watched you kill yourself so that you could prove a point. I'm behind you either way, but I want you to ask yourself if this is what God would have you do. Would He have you quit?"

Her words were piercing. I knew they were true, but I still couldn't handle them; and I wanted to give up. I just didn't have enough courage to face the stage that night.

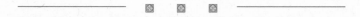

In an effort to prevent me from making what she knew would be a tragic decision, Kendra suggested I call Darren and Deke to get their opinions. My first call was to Darren, who blasted me for even considering not showing up to the finals. "Who cares how big the other guys are?" he asked. "You did the best you could, and that's all we wanted from the start. We worked our backsides off for this, so I'll see you later."

Then came my call to Deke. And his lecture was one that has burned in me ever since.

"Who are you doing this for?" he asked. "Is this really about how great you look or who you can beat tonight? No. This is about a man who, through his faith, pushed past every obstacle to be able to compete today. It doesn't matter what you look like or what the other guys look like. You're not really competing against anyone else today, brother; you're competing against yourself, and you've already won. I'm proud of you; Darren is proud of you; Kendra is proud of you; and God is proud of you. I'll see you at 5:00 p.m."

With all the support and a little kick in the butt, my pity party came to an end. Kendra was right. So were Darren and Deke. Was I really going to throw all the months of pain, perseverance, sacrifice, dedication, and faith away because of pride? That would have been a slap in the face to God. He'd shown me unbelievable favor, blessed me with strength when what I was doing wasn't humanly possible, and provided me with more encouraging supporters than I deserved. He'd deepened my relationship with Him and answered too many of my prayers. Quitting was not an option.

———————— ▦ ▦ ▦ ————————

I rested a little while that afternoon and then headed back to Dr. Phillips High School for the finals. Kendra drove as I shoveled carbs into my mouth in order to help me fill out, but it didn't seem to be working. Contest dieting is a science, and I was such a unique case that all we could do was guess. Right now my whole timing, calorie intake, and food ratios were off and I didn't seem to be responding to the carbs.

Even if I wasn't in trophy contention, I was still set on looking the best I could for the individual posing routine.

The auditorium entrance was a mob scene, and Kendra and I had to push passed the crowd to get inside. It was obvious that we were going to have a packed house. We found Kendra a seat as close to the front as possible, and I went backstage to meet Darren and get ready.

Jim and Tina were once again waiting there to help me get oiled and pumped up. Mike Ives also spotted me and came over, as did several others. A few of the athletes who hadn't said anything to me earlier that morning began introducing themselves, and most of them stopped their prep work to talk with me. It was evident that someone—whether Deke, Ives, or someone else—had explained who I was and what I was doing.

The admiration these guys showed me was amazing. They hugged me, shook my hand, and told me how inspired they were. Right then I knew it would have been a horrible mistake to quit. It was clear that the MS Bodybuilding Challenge was worth it, if only to bring hope, faith, and inspiration to others. If I'd given in to fear and pride, I would have bailed out of a once-in-a-lifetime opportunity to change lives. Thank God He'd rescued me once more and delivered me to the contest.

When the contest began, we separated into our classes, lined up by number, and walked on stage for the mandatory poses. The guys in line with me could see that it wasn't easy for me, and they supported me as we made our way out. The process was exhilarating, and I could feel the competitor in me start to come alive. The battle against myself and my disease was being waged, and the good side was winning. We posed as a group, left the stage, and waited for the individual routines to be called.

Darren's class had already gone through the finals by the time mine was up. While he looked cut and muscular and was in fantastic condition, he didn't place where he wanted. He placed fifth in the over-forty class, and my condolences to him made us both laugh when I joked, "At least you don't have MS."

Finally it was time for my class to come out and pose individually to our selected music. Right before I stepped out in front of the standing-room-only crowd, the emcee took a moment to tell my story. He talked about courage and determination and how no one had ever stepped on stage with MS in that contest before. I felt emotion well up inside of me that begged to overflow. I wanted to savor the moment and embrace what was taking place: on August 22, 2009, at the age of fifty and with MS, I was standing on stage competing with more than 150 healthy athletes in the Florida State Bodybuilding Championships.

As I walked out onto the stage, I felt God's anointing on my life—His purpose His will. The song I had chosen for the routine was "Fighter" by Christina Aguilera. The lyrics of the chorus seemed to accurately fit my situation, as I felt like I had been a fighter against MS all along. While it meant to do me harm, the disease had actually made me stronger and wiser and had made my skin thicker. I had become a new breed of warrior in a battle I'd never anticipated. But I was grateful—thankful that God had made me a fighter.

I began my routine and experienced some difficulty holding each pose and keeping my balance, but I was determined to get through it as smoothly as possible. The world seemed to stop during those two and a half minutes. It was me and God, and nothing more.

The spotlights kept me from seeing the crowd below, but I could hear their cheers and applause as I went through my poses. I knew my routine well, and because Kendra had made me practice several times a day for weeks leading up to the contest, I struck each one on cue. Even though I wasn't massive, insanely ripped, or perfectly symmetrical, and I was flexing with only a fraction of a right pec, the crowd still erupted after certain poses. Kendra, who had been out there proudly making sure everyone knew I was her husband, later told me that they gave me a standing ovation.

When the music ended, I felt a rush of relief that it was finally over. I was truly exhausted and could feel an MS flare-up coming on, and it took all of my remaining strength to control the shaking in my left leg. I knew I needed to get out of the spotlight, but I wanted to live in that moment forever. I felt God's presence surrounding me, and I stood tall as I walked off stage still hearing the cheering.

After the remaining competitors in my class were finished, I heard the emcee calling my name again. Because it was so noisy backstage with weights clanging and everyone shuffling to get ready for their routines, I never quite heard what he said. As I stood there wiping off the oil and getting ready to get dressed, Deke rushed over to me and ushered me back on stage. He'd told me in our phone conversation that morning that he had something planned for me, but I had no idea what to expect. I was about to find out.

Once I was back on stage, the emcee announced that I was the winner of the Most Inspirational Bodybuilder trophy. I couldn't believe it. Again the crowd erupted and stood to give me an ovation. It turned out that I would be going home with a prize after all. I accepted the trophy and walked off the stage, knowing that this trophy meant more than anything I could have won for physical performance.

Backstage, Darren, Jim, Tina, Deke, and Ives were waiting to congratulate me. I shook hands, gave hugs, and embraced the moment with my amazing support team. Still, nothing felt so great as when I reunited with Kendra, who hugged me and told me she was proud of me.

To have a wife who had supported my dreams and goals was a trophy in and of itself.

———————————— ▨ ◈ ▨ ————————————

Before we left I paused for a few moments to look around. I soaked in the atmosphere—the mess of weights, the towels on the floor, and the gym bags—and inhaled the blended scent of posing oil and tanning spray. I briefly closed my eyes and was taken back twenty-five years to when I didn't have MS and was a young man. But right then, those factors didn't matter to me like they had that morning. I was a new competitor—a stronger one in many ways. I thanked the Lord for giving me the strength to overcome every obstacle that had been thrown in my path on the road to victory. I opened my eyes and took one last look around before we packed up and all left the auditorium together.

Chapter 9

GOD USES GREAT PEOPLE

The day after the contest was a day of reflection. It marked the beginning of a new chapter in my life, and I spent time pondering what had just taken place and wondering what was ahead. The MS Bodybuilding Challenge had been a success, and God had carried me every step of the way. Now, with this goal accomplished, it was time to make some decisions about the future.

My children had always been my priority, which was why Kendra and I had stayed in the Celebration area. I loved being able to see them often, and I didn't want to be away from them for a moment. But from where we were geographically, it was becoming increasingly difficult to conduct business in the entertainment industry.

While there were many production companies in Florida that produce TV shows and films, the most successful ones were based in Los Angeles, California, and there was no way around it. One local company called Pink Sneakers, which had been successful through shows such as *Hogan Knows Best*, had been working with me on a deal for a show I'd created, but it wasn't moving in the direction I had hoped, so there was really no long-term business relationship that was keeping us in Florida. In fact, Kendra and I were now flying back and forth to LA for meetings with companies that did want to do business with me, but the distance was hindering all of the deals. It was time to make the move out west—both for business and for Kendra, who would enjoy being back home. We started making plans and decided to move after the first of the year in 2010.

The one thing that made leaving difficult was having to say good-bye to friends.

It's funny. People occasionally ask me the question, "If you could change your life and not have MS, would you?" To me, that's not really worth answering. I've been dealt these cards, and I have to work with what I have. Worrying about things I can't change is a waste of time. Instead, I focus on what MS has given me, instead. It has allowed me to touch the lives of others, to show people my heart, to reach people for Christ, and to expand my circle of friends and meet some of the most amazing men and women on the planet.

How could I say good-bye to guys like Darren, Jim, and Deke and so many others who had become such a big part of my life? Still, it was time to depart. Both Kendra and I agreed, and we felt God's leading in the new direction.

So, with our little dog Kammie in tow, we drove across the country to set up our new life in California.

It was February 2010 when we arrived. After we settled into our townhome in Thousand Oaks—a suburb just northwest of LA—Kendra went back to work as a home health nurse while I worked on Lyons Entertainment. I was still involved with *Hog Heaven*, but it was only airing reruns, and we weren't in new production for another season. I needed to find my way back into the development and production of new TV shows.

When we arrived, I was blessed to learn that the one friendly connection I had in the business was going to help me get started. A woman I had met through meetings wanted me to come work for her company, so I contacted her and began working with her on projects. That proved to be a great way to develop inroads, but it wasn't going to help build Lyons Entertainment, and I needed to focus on developing my own business. I kept seeking work in other areas, believing that God had a plan that He would reveal in His time.

With my focus narrowed to business, I found myself missing the challenge of bodybuilding competition. I hadn't stopped training hard, but I wanted to compete again someday, and it was clear that I was in the right environment. As home to some of the best amateur and professional bodybuilders in the world, Southern California has gyms located every few miles. Training wouldn't be a problem. Driving, however, would be a different story.

Because of an episode I'd experienced in Florida, in which I'd lost all feeling in my arm and almost crashed our car, Kendra didn't like me driving. And with my occasional loss of vision in my left eye and the threat of double-vision, it was safer for me to rely on Kendra to be my chauffeur. Any workouts I would do would have to revolve around her work schedule.

I started training six days a week while working on Lyons Entertainment from home. Kendra drove me wherever I needed to go, whether to meetings or to the gym, and for a while she even trained with me. But, because I am a bit intense, slightly impatient, and occasionally self-absorbed while at the gym, she decided to work out on her own. To this day she teases me that she can hear my grunting from across the gym.

I was on my own in the training this time, but I was still getting advice from Darren and others from thousands of miles away. Because I wanted to compete again, I kept a high level of training intensity. I wasn't about to enter my next contest looking small or being dwarfed by the competition. Next time I wanted a chance to place; so, until I selected a contest, my goal became to get as big as I could.

——————————— ▣   ▣   ▣ ———————————

As much as multiple sclerosis hindered my ability to train, it also crippled certain aspects of my daily life. The level of fatigue it brought impaired my ability to work on business as hard and as long as I wanted. I easily lost the ability to concentrate throughout the day, and by dinner time I was brain dead. My coordination faded, and I struggled to walk a straight line or lift my legs to climb a flight of stairs.

For me, though, the most frustrating part was how nonstop I had been prior to the first attack. From my days as a gym owner in my twenties and thirties to my stock-trading years, I had always woken up early, gone to bed late, and never stopped thinking. As an MS patient, I was no longer an Energizer Bunny who could keep going and going. I felt more like the tortoise in his race against the hare. I would eventually get there and win, but it would take me a heck of a long time.

If I'd been able to get a full night's sleep once in a while, it would have helped combat the fatigue, but that wasn't happening. Regardless of how much I tried to sleep, the MS would keep me awake. It wasn't just from the pins-and-needles feeling, it was from the pain in my body and the strange tremors that affected my sleep pattern. My anxiety was also growing, as I would wonder whether tomorrow would be the day I'd experience another exacerbation. I spent many hours at night praying that God would keep the disease from advancing, and poor Kendra would often be woken up by me getting out of bed to try and walk off the MS feeling or calm my anxiety.

Studies have shown that the uncertainty of the symptoms, the progression, and the exacerbation episodes make MS one of the most difficult diseases to handle psychologically. No one likes the unknown, and it is a disease that revolves around it.

I hated having MS. And I hated that it could and would be worsened by stress, heat, overworking, and—well, just about anything.

Here's how the National MS Society explains exacerbations:

> It can be very mild or severe enough to interfere with a person's ability to function at home and at work. No two exacerbations are alike, and symptoms vary from person to person and from one exacerbation to another. For example, the exacerbation might be an episode of optic neuritis (caused by inflammation of the optic nerve that impairs vision) or problems with balance or severe fatigue. Some relapses produce only one symptom (related to inflammation in a single area of the central nervous system) while other relapses cause two or more symptoms at the same time (related to inflammation in more than one area of the central nervous system).
>
> To be a true exacerbation, the attack must last at least 24 hours and be separated from the previous attack by at least 30 days. Most exacerbations last from a few days to several weeks or even months.

Exacerbations are caused by inflammation in the central nervous system. The inflammation damages the myelin, which slows or disrupts the transmission of nerve impulses and causes the symptoms of MS.

In the most common disease course in MS—called relapsing-remitting MS—clearly defined acute exacerbations (relapses) are followed by remissions as the inflammatory process gradually comes to an end. Going into remission doesn't necessarily mean that the symptoms disappear totally—some people will return to feeling exactly as they did before the exacerbation began while others may find themselves left with some ongoing symptoms. ("Exacerbations," www.nationalmssociety.org)

To me, living with the disease of the unknown was like living in a black hole and constantly trying to find my way to the light. It was a 24/7 problem, and all of the MS limitations were tormenting me. I never knew what tomorrow—or even later that day—would bring regarding symptoms; and I really didn't know how to deal with it other than to pray, ask for healing, and have faith like I'd always done. And occasionally that was a challenge in itself.

The best thing I could do was to focus outward and put my attention on helping and inspiring others, which was something I missed after the MS Bodybuilding Challenge ended. I again reached out to the Fellowship of Christian Athletes to write devotionals and speak whenever I could; and as I built Lyons Entertainment and worked out at the gym, I took every opportunity I had to tell my story and let everyone know that God was my strength. I set my sights on Christ and forged ahead.

By this time, I had started to realize how much God had changed me. Through His Word and staying connected with Him during such an intense season of life and the MS Bodybuilding Challenge, I discovered that I had come to a place of intimacy with Him that I'd never experienced before. It's funny how that works. In fact, it's funny how a lot of things work with God.

Walking with Him at all can become a puzzling, confusing, and frustrating journey if we let it. There are times when we've all wanted to ask God, "Why me?" when faced with adversity, but I was learning to start asking a different question instead: "Lord, what is my purpose in this trial?"

Whenever we start to wonder why God has allowed our obstacles, we need to look back to His Word and find the answer.

In Romans 8:36 we read that, as followers of Christ, we are considered "as sheep to be slaughtered." Now, that would be a very scary statement if that's where it ended. If all we had to look forward to were life's adversities, we would never be able to endure.

Many times along my journey, I felt hopelessness threaten to settle in and make its home in my soul. But in those times, I had to consciously make an effort to change my thoughts and focus on God's truth—that He had a good plan and an ultimate purpose.

To me, part of that involves knowing that as sheep to be slaughtered we aren't just animals without faith, being led unknowingly to death. We are children of God, our good Shepherd, being led purposefully into life. Part of that journey involves enduring suffering. And our faith during those times allows Him to make us fruitful, especially in the eyes of those who doubt. As His followers, it is our duty to show the world that, through obstacles, hardship, disease, poverty, and whatever else we may face, we walk in the footsteps of a Mighty God who can make a path, even in the "valley of the shadow of death" (Ps. 23:4).

In Genesis 41:52, Joseph proclaims that God made him fruitful in the land of his suffering. And I've learned that this is what our trials are for: generating His glory. In fact, God produced the greatest fruit of all time—our salvation—out of the greatest suffering of all time—Christ on the cross.

If we stood face to face with Jesus today and asked Him if He liked the trials He endured to save our souls, I doubt He would say yes. While I'm sure He had a certain level of joy, it didn't mean He had to like the process. It would have been far easier for Him to have been on a journey in which everyone loved Him, listened to Him and accepted Him, but the results wouldn't have been the same. Because He endured adversity that no mere human could have endured, He achieved the amazing end result of our salvation and the payment for our sins.

Through my own suffering, I came to realize that it didn't really matter whether I suffered in life because I would be treated to everlasting life in the presence of God in the end. My goal while here on earth was to allow God to use my trials in order to bring His truth and love to the world so that others could put their faith in Him and join Him in heaven, too. None of us are here for the satisfaction of our flesh, but to be of service to God. Once we truly understand that, accept it, and choose to endure whatever we must in order to be in the will of God, our trials will no longer be trials but walks of faith.

On my journey, I also was learning that God has a way of challenging and increasing my faith with each increasing level of adversity. I didn't like the fact that I had multiple sclerosis—I still don't—but I embraced the challenge as a means of exemplifying the power of God and His grace in my life. I was here to be a testimony to His great love by overcoming what some would call a catastrophic situation.

While I will never claim that I can perfectly view it this way, I do know that MS has been a gift in many ways. Through the disease, I was able to embrace more of my identity in Christ and discover my true purpose here on earth. I was a willing believer who would take the journey with God through any suffering and obstacles that needed be endured for His glory.

⊞   ⊞   ⊞

As the days wore on, I became more willing to accept God's strength in the trial of MS. I viewed it as a test of faith and a test of myself, and through it miraculous things continued to happen for me in California.

Through a God-ordained "coincidence," I received a call from a producer who offered me a chance to work with him on a reality show project. I accepted his offer, and that connection led me to a woman in the finance industry who thought what I was accomplishing, not only in bodybuilding but also in the entertainment business, was nothing short of astonishing. In March of that year, she arranged a phone call with a man in the TV production business whom she thought would be a possible collaboration partner for me. His name was Andrew Bishop, and he had been working in the production side of entertainment with top companies, such as CBS, for more than twenty years.

On our call, Andrew and I both felt at ease with each other, and this led us to set up an in-person meeting. When we met, we discussed possible projects and landed on one that seemed to be a perfect fit. We also got to know each other on a personal level and discovered that we shared a mutual faith. In fact, Andrew had been baptized by Rick Warren, the founder and pastor of Saddleback Church in California and one of the most influential pastors in America. We both could see that God was doing something through our connection, so we planned to work together and start the development and production of what is called a sizzle reel, which we could use to pitch our show to networks.

As part of the partnership, Andrew brought along his wife, Lane—an Emmy Award–winning director—and a team of the most creative people I had ever met, which included John Spagnola and Kendall Lamkin, two incredibly talented young men. During the shoot, Andrew, Lane, the team, and I jelled immediately. It was like we had worked together for years. Even Kendra, whom I'd recruited as a production assistant for Lane, fit right in and was such a trooper. She'd never worked production before and was doing the work on her day off from nursing.

From production to editing, everything went smoothly, and Andrew and I realized an opportunity to form a long-term partnership. As it turned out, the guy I met through a "chance" connection turned out to be the man who is now my greatest business partner and best friend. We merged our two companies and have since built Bishop-Lyons Entertainment (BLE). It's risen up from a small company based out of Andrew's house to one that has offices in LA and partnerships with some of TV's biggest agents, producers, and production companies. All of this happened within a year of our working together.

It's hard for me to express how much of a blessing Andrew was and continues to be. To this day he picks up the slack when the MS takes its toll on me, and everyone—Lane; John, our vice president of postproduction, and Kendall, our director of postproduction—helps keep the company running like clockwork, while I work from home doing business over the phone. It is a group of "I have your back" people that only God could have assembled. My job is to keep the business income flowing, and theirs is to produce the highest level of content available. This kind of connection on a team is rare, and yet we have it. I don't mind using the word miraculous, because I believe everything God does is of that magnitude, and I know it's the case with our group. They have even supported my bodybuilding challenge, and, thanks to them, I have a redesigned MS Bodybuilding Challenge website and new video promos for the cause. Now, not only are we working to produce great entertainment projects, we are collectively partnering to help MS patients throughout the world.

In July 2010, I was excited to be contacted by a man named Marty Jacobus, the multi-area director for FCA in that part of Southern California. He'd heard about me through Jimmy Page and wanted me to start speaking at events. Soon, Marty gave me the opportunity to share my personal testimony in front of high school students in my area. I continued contributing to FCA's daily email devotions and was even honored to be asked to write several for their 2011 Athlete's Bible. It was incredibly important to me to continue sharing what God had done and continued to do in my life in the face of MS.

As I watched God deliver blessing after blessing to me, I started to really examine my heart and re-evaluate the purpose of the MS Bodybuilding Challenge. Honestly, I had lost a little perspective. Thankfully, I was married to a woman who wasn't afraid to speak the truth. In a very pointed discussion, Kendra put my feet to the fires of perspective and asked, "Dave, are you just doing this so that you can overcome MS for yourself, or are you using this to help others?"

I really had to think. My heart was truly in the right place, but I could feel that there was conviction taking place. Yes, I was inspiring people with and without MS, preaching the Lord's gospel, and being a role model for youth, but was I helping others like me? That was the question Kendra brought to my attention. Was I focusing so much on training and on getting big for another contest that I was missing a major opportunity from the Lord? This would take some prayer.

Through a true heart examination, I realized that I had somehow convinced myself that all I needed to do was compete again in order for the world to be a better place for those who had MS. So I prayed, "Lord, is the MS Bodybuilding Challenge my challenge alone, or do I need to change the focus? Am I in Your will or in my own? Is my ego getting the best of me?" As I kept praying for His guidance, it came.

In the three years since I'd begun the MS Bodybuilding Challenge, I'd received many emails and phone calls from those who had told me how much I'd inspired them. I had been featured on TV and radio shows and had been written about in books and articles. All of this had certainly been enough to make me proud of myself and send my ego through the roof. And, the more that was accomplished, the easier it became for me to feed my pride.

I am human, and I sometimes forget what's really going on. I forget that it is God at work, not David, and I start taking credit for it when all the while it has been Christ who led the way and supplied the might and power for the venture. Everything I was able to do had been through His strength. If it had been up to me, I would have collapsed like one of the mountains God could crumble. One of the most humbling verses I read at that time was Habakkuk 3:6: "He stood, and shook the earth; he looked, and made the nations tremble. The ancient mountains crumbled and the age-old hills collapsed. His ways are eternal." He was the strong One, not me.

The Lord warns us in Scripture that walking in pride is not a godly course of action. In fact, it leads to our downfall. As a Christian and an ambassador for Christ, I knew in my heart that I needed to focus on Him and remember that I was His representative to those watching. Selfish pride had no place in my life, and in all of the triumphs I needed to be serving as the light of the Lord, radiating His humility and love. With Kendra's loving nudge, I realized that my focus had gotten off track.

—————————— ▣ ▣ ▣ ——————————

In John 15:5, Jesus says that apart from Him we can do nothing. There is no strength in our humanness. There are no victories without Him, either in bodybuilding or in general life. When we are champions, we are to be champions for Him in order to reveal Him to the world and display His power. When we look in our mirrors, we need to see ourselves as vessels through which God can do His will.

When I saw what was going on in my heart, I knew I needed to make a change. I didn't want ego, pride, or selfishness to stand in the way of my being in God's will. So, with His voice in my soul and Kendra's voice in my ear, I stood up to my ego and pride and set out to achieve higher goals, but ones rooted in His grace, love, and power. I desperately wanted to be a warrior for Christ instead of for myself, and for Him to be the ultimate Champion of the MS Bodybuilding Challenge.

At that moment, I realized that even when we are doing good we need to periodically re-evaluate our motives and rediscover the root issues of our purpose. Why are we pushing forward? If it's not for God's ultimate glory, something needs to change. For me, that time was now.

—————————— ▣ ▣ ▣ ——————————

Shortly after this awakening, I was in the gym training when I heard a few guys talking about how they were going to compete in a bodybuilding contest one day. *Hmmm*, I thought to myself. *How many times have I heard people talking about what they are going to do "one day"?* Too many times. I'd heard so many people say what they dreamed of doing only to never follow through.

For me, that is a tragedy, and I have personally made it a goal to not let myself fall into that category. In my fifty-plus years, I've come to believe that, when I talk about accomplishing a task that I believe to be in line with God's will, He expects me to follow through.

When Jesus talked about doing something, He did it. He made no empty promises, and He always kept His word. Through personal experience and my relationship with Him, I've found that He still operates that way. As His followers, then, and as those who are called to imitate Him, we should follow His example and carry out whatever we say we will do. Obviously this doesn't include sinful action, but if we have discerned that Christ is leading us to pursue a certain goal, we must be faithful to carry it out instead of merely talking about it.

When I heard these guys in the gym I turned to them and quoted 1 Corinthians 4:20: "For the kingdom of God is not a matter of talk but of power." I explained to them that words without actions were empty and that it was the power of the Holy Spirit we needed in order to accomplish our goals.

At first, they looked at me like I had three eyes, but when I told them what God had done in my life through the MS Bodybuilding Challenge, their mouths dropped open and the looks on their faces changed. Now I had their attention. That day, God showed both them and me a powerful lesson. He spoke His Truth to the men in the gym, and He also allowed me to see the platform and power He had given me through my testimony.

"This is the word of the LORD to Zerubbabel: 'Not by might nor by power, but by my Spirit,' says the LORD Almighty" (Zech. 4:6). Much like John 15:5, this verse illustrates that it is not our own power that propels us to success; it is God's. As believers, we are to follow in His footsteps and let His power fuel our talk. I could see in their eyes that these young men left the gym that day wanting what I had received from my relationship with Christ. Who wouldn't want the kind of power that could raise the dead?

When I got home, I looked back and carefully examined what I had told the men. I realized that this was one way God was going to use my battle against MS to influence others. It dawned on me that although I was following through with God's plan to battle this disease in a unique way though bodybuilding, I wasn't doing all I could to help others beat it as well. I had been talking about how I was helping MS patients, but I hadn't been carrying out that part of the mission.

In an attempt to maximize the effort, Kendra and I developed a new plan and shared it with Andrew. We told him that we needed to do more for MS patients by adding a new element to the MS Bodybuilding Challenge. This new aspect wouldn't be as much about bodybuilding as it would be about fitness and the importance of getting their bodies to move. If I could challenge people with MS to embrace physical activity and to take care of themselves through a healthy diet and positive mindset, I could help them live a more full and vibrant life.

No one would have to compete in a bodybuilding contest. We knew that those who had been in wheelchairs for years or who were using walkers weren't going to be inspired to go out and lift a thousand pounds with their legs anytime soon. There wouldn't be any requirement to enter a competition or follow in my footsteps. In all honesty, I don't recommend this kind of training for others. The MS Bodybuilding Challenge was my personal way of overcoming the obstacle and slaying my Goliath, but it was an extremely draining way to beat the odds and one that caused a variety of injuries. It should certainly not be the standard for fighting MS. However, a solid regimen of health and fitness should be.

◈   ◈   ◈

With the new desire to encourage other MS patients toward healthy lives, we officially launched the MS Fitness Challenge. As a bodybuilder, I would be the spokesperson, but my goal would now be to reach out to those with MS and help them to do all they could to fight the disease.

Andrew and the rest of our company stood behind this plan of action and began working to promote the cause through video promotions and our website. Kendra and I also met with the National MS Society, and we started working together to make the MS Fitness Challenge an ongoing program. It's been a monumental undertaking that has taken a tremendous amount of planning, money, time, and support, but we're all committed to banding together and forging ahead. It is our hope that, through this adventure, others who share my condition will be inspired to live beyond the chains of this disease and realize that they have the power to break them. It is a power not their own, but one from a source greater than any on this earth.

I can do everything through him who gives me strength.
(Phil. 4:13)

Chapter 10

ONE MORE TIME

In stark contrast to the previous few years, 2011 passed quickly with no major setbacks in training, no injuries, and nothing new in regards to MS symptoms. They seemed to have stabilized at the level of no feeling in my left arm and hand—other than pins, needles, and tightness—limited coordination and movement in my left leg, and the occasional exacerbation. Bishop-Lyons Entertainment had grown tremendously, and we had deals in place with many major companies including Triage Entertainment, which produced the Food Network's *Iron Chef*, and 3 Ball Productions, who handled NBC's hit *The Biggest Loser*. We had also sold a show to Animal Planet, and things were going well with Andrew handling the office and patiently supporting my MS goals, and Lane, John, and Kendall forming our core team.

Thanks to Andrew's support in watching over the business, I had the chance to speak at several FCA high school "Huddle" meetings. Kendra always came with me and served as my biggest advocate and cheerleader. With everything that was going on in my life and the level of MS-caused exhaustion, I felt that it was important to keep fighting to demonstrate that the Lord came first.

At these Huddle meetings, I would tell my story to the young men and women in the audience and recount how the Lord had worked in my life and my disease-filled body. Many times, I would look out into the audience and question whether they were really listening and taking in what I was saying or just daydreaming. What I discovered was that they were part of FCA because they loved the Lord and wanted to soak in everything they could to develop their relationships with Him. Most of them sat with eyes wide open as I spoke, applauded when I was finished, and asked great questions at the end, letting me know they had truly been paying attention.

At these Huddle meetings, I also got to see just how much everyone loves Kendra—and with good reason. She is the softness to my hardness, and her bubbly personality allows her to bond easily with people in a crowd. In the back of my mind, I always wonder whether people who meet us are asking themselves how such a sweet woman can deal with such a rough man. But I know the answer. She sees right through my tough exterior and into my heart. And, as we both continued to praise God and tell others of His work in our lives, I could see and feel His hand at work in both of us.

⸺⸺⸺ ◈ ◈ ◈ ⸺⸺⸺

The goal to compete again was imbedded in me, and I was training hard and eating close to five thousand calories a day. I wasn't restricting carbs, was eating healthy fats, and had put on a lot of body weight. I felt like the time was right for me to do it all again and enter another con-test—to begin the countdown to my next competition as a bodybuilder with multiple sclerosis.

At age fifty-three, I was a few years older than I had been when I'd last competed, and it certainly wasn't getting any easier. But by this time, I knew that the Lord would supply all the strength I needed to keep pushing on and battle this disease—and win. This time around, I had a clearer vision of His purpose than I did in 2008, and it continues to take shape with each day that passes. Now I know that, without a doubt, it is my calling to help others with MS use fitness in order to battle their disease and defeat their own Goliaths. I want everyone to embrace God's available victory and to tap into His power. "The Lord will march out like a champion, like a warrior he will stir up his zeal; with a shout he will raise the battle cry and will triumph over his enemies" (Isa. 42:13).

In a sport filled with healthy young men, I'll always be the under-dog. I'll always be the one who, in theory, shouldn't be on that stage. I'm not just battling weights; I'm battling the threat of being placed in a wheelchair. My competition isn't just the guys next to me, it's the shaking in my legs and the all-consuming exhaustion—the pins and needles and constant threat of injury. But, with the incredible support of so many friends, family, and professionals, and with the Lord supply-ing the power and strength, I will continue this bodybuilding journey until I hear Him say it's enough. And I just don't see that happening anytime soon.

———————————— ▣ ▣ ▣ ————————————

As I started this new chapter of my battle against MS, God led some amazing new people into my life. People like John Lepak, the head of advertising at Powerhouse Gym International and a wonderful Christian man, and Krystal Dabish, the director of business relations for the company, both of whom got behind the MS Bodybuilding Challenge and MS Fitness Challenge. With more than three hundred locations worldwide, Powerhouse Gym has almost two million members, and their company has been a huge supporter of my cause and given me so many opportunities to promote it and help others. They have printed articles about the Challenge in their magazine and featured me on their website as a way of bringing awareness to MS.

Another great relationship started in 2011 when fitness author, motivational speaker, and radio/TV personality John Rowley joined my fight. I met him at the Powerhouse Gym convention in Las Vegas, and he has stayed by my side ever since. As both a friend and colleague, he's helped me in so many ways, and, as a successful author himself with Leafwood Publishers, he was the first to suggest that they publish this book. John has hosted me on his fitness radio show and his Christian TV show, and he is now hosting a radio show called MS Fitness Mondays with the National MS Society, which I am underwriting.

As a brother in Christ, John is a ceaseless blessing to me. He and I were both gym owners in the old days, and, because he is a fellow fifty-something bodybuilder, he and I speak the same language. Even though we live across the country from one another, John and I were able to work out together once when I was doing TV production in his area of North Carolina. I know I can speak for John when I say we both felt like we were still in our twenties as we pushed through that workout. Whenever we'd pass by the mirrors, we'd look at our reflections and wonder who the old guys were!

One way that many of these new relationships were being established was through sponsorships. Mark Webb, the owner of the nutritional supplement company High Energy Labs, supplied me with supplements that have helped me sleep better, avoid joint pain, and increase my growth hormone levels, which is a necessity in developing muscle and slowing down the aging process. His products have also helped with my MS symptoms, and there's no way I could thank him enough for that.

Because he's developed a passion for the cause, Mark is also helping Andrew and me launch the supplement line in Bishop-Lyons Entertainment's new fitness brand called NaturalBody. It may sound strange for an entertainment company to be creating a supplement line, but it's actually a natural with my fitness background to launch a fitness division.

Through NaturalBody, we produce fitness DVDs, TV shows, supplements, web support, and resources for the health and wellness market, focusing on baby boomers—including those with disabilities—who need guidance in health and fitness. It's yet another way we can impact other by helping them uncover a rich, vibrant life.

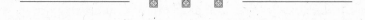

Throughout the journey, I've also met many fitness trainers who have helped me by sending new workouts and training ideas my way; their help has been a blessing. One trainer I was reunited with after thirty years was Mike Torchia, a one-time Teenage Mr. America and, years later, Mr. California.

I knew Mike from my gym days in New York when he was a few years older and already making a lot of noise in the amateur competition circle. At the time, I was living in Queens, New York, and I regularly drove forty-five minutes to Long Island in order to train at Mr. America's Gym, which was the mecca of bodybuilding in the area, similar to what Gold's is in California. But there was another gym that was much closer to me in Brooklyn that was *the* place to go. It was called

R&J Health Studio, and it was where the Incredible Hulk himself, Lou Ferrigno, trained.

Unlike Mr. America's, R&J was a very small gym, and it was easy to run into champions there. This gym was where scenes from the infamous movie *Pumping Iron* were filmed and where my friend John Rowley would later become owner.

Instead of driving all the way out to Long Island, I would sometimes just go from Queens to Brooklyn to get in a workout at R&J's, and that's where I met Mike, who was actually training with Lou at the time. Despite his reputation as an intense, bar-bending bodybuilder, Mike was friendly. Back then, he was trying to make his mark in the sport and was working out hard, but he still took the time to talk to me and encourage me.

After he left New York, Mike moved to California, where he won the Mr. California title and became a celebrity fitness trainer, working with stars such as Al Pacino and Matt Damon. While I hadn't seen or been in touch with Mike since New York, I'd heard much about him and what he was doing. Bodybuilding has many athletes all over the world, but it is still a small circle; and one day, while John Rowley was speaking to Mike, he asked him if he knew me and about the MS Bodybuilding Challenge. After all those years, Mike did remember me, and he quickly gave me a call.

Mike and I spoke at length, reminiscing about the past and telling stories; and, after our long conversation, he offered to help in any way he could. Since then, he has connected me to a great sports medicine doctor, Dr. Rand McClain, and a chiropractor, Jason Kelberman, who both work with MS patients and understand the challenges of bodybuilding with this disease. Mike has helped support the MS Bodybuilding Challenge and the MS Fitness Challenge, and he has given me a great deal of training and nutritional advice. His knowledge is vast, and his desire to help is great. He's there when I need him and is always willing to do what he can to assist me.

Mike has been a gift from God, and I count him and all of the others as unbelievable blessings. In Romans 8:28, we read that in all things God works for the good of those who love Him and who have been called by Him. Through all of these relationships and connections, I have seen that truth at work. Not only is God working to bless others through this challenge, He's also blessing me with friends and team-mates and increasing my physical, emotional, and spiritual strength. The relationships have been every bit as important as all of the weights and training. It has truly all worked for good.

With such a strong support team, I still desired to connect with others who could relate to my specific situation. Like I said before, it's so dif-ficult to explain the symptoms of MS in a way that makes sense to someone who has never experienced them. When I feel like my body is vibrating from the inside out or the numbness is running through my extremities, does anyone understand? What about the constant, tight pins and needles that I experience when I try to close my left hand? Can anyone imagine how that feels? And those are just the constant symptoms. There are also ones that come and go from day to day or even hour by hour, and it's impossible to really get it if you've never experienced them.

That's why I enjoy talking to other MS patients. It's encouraging to be able to refer to a symptom and have someone say, "Yeah, I have that one too." I don't need to elaborate; they just get it. It's incredibly refreshing when I'm so used to seeing people stare at me in confusion.

While I'm sharing frustrations and being honest, I will add one more. At the gym, people see me as a big, strong man training alongside twenty- and thirty-year-old bodybuilders, and they have no idea what I'm battling because I look just fine. While I want it that way, I sometimes wish they really knew what was going on. It's a battle that is partly driven by pride and that is partly spiritual in nature.

The prideful side of me wants people to pat me on the back and say, "Wow, I can't believe you're doing that in your condition." But the other part of me—the Holy Spirit side—wants people to know how hard it is so that they can see the power of God at work. Yes, I look the part when I train—praise God! But it can be frustrating not to feel like anyone around me sees that, and it's just one more thing I'll have to leave in God's hands. And as for the pride, that remains an area of struggle for me, and I lose many battles with it. But I'll never stop fighting.

Still, God redeems even His sin-filled sons and daughters, giving them testimonies through situations like I experienced one morning not long ago.

I woke up at 5:00 A.M. experiencing severe MS symptoms, and all I could do was sit with the pain, numbness, and pins and needles. I could barely get my legs to coordinate enough to walk up and down the stairs, and I was shaking uncontrollably. At 11:00 a.m., I was scheduled to do a radio interview with John Rowley to talk about the MS Bodybuilding Challenge and how my faith had played a role in it all. To be honest, my faith wasn't at an all-time high at the moment, and I wasn't sure I could pretend that everything was fine. Still, I prayed for strength, dug in, counted my blessings, and went to the interview. It was an act of will, obedience, and devotion to the Lord, who had called me to share about His work in my life.

When the show began, I was still in severe pain; but over the course of our interview, the symptoms, which had lasted for six hours, diminished in a mere thirty minutes. It was a truly humbling experience. By acting in faith and not giving in to my flesh—by carrying out the Lord's will instead of my own—He showed me that His strength would give me mine. It was powerful and encouraging to feel His hand relieving my pain, and it further increased my resolve to persevere both through and for Him.

I go through those bouts of severe pain often, but I seldom complain. Mainly, I don't want Kendra to know how I'm feeling. I worry that it will scare her, so I keep it to myself. Sometimes, though, it gets so bad that it even scares me.

Living in this body can be almost unbearable. I try my best to block it out, get business done, and train, but I get tired of fighting MS every day. I get weary of not knowing whether tomorrow will be the day I have to stop walking. I hate living with the symptoms, waiting for them to subside, and always worrying this will be the time that they won't.

It breaks my heart when I feel this way in light of all the great things in my life. I've been blessed with the ultimate gift of a wonderful wife, who married me even knowing I had MS; but I also see the limits that MS has set around us. As determined as I am to fight this disease, I know there are certain realities.

I know Kendra would like to go dancing with her husband, but I don't have the coordination to do it. I know my children would like to see me more in Florida, but I can't sit on a plane without extreme pain. I have the desire to work tirelessly at my business, yet MS exhausts me halfway through the day.

If I allowed myself to do it, I could go on and on about how MS puts a damper on many of life's experiences. There are many days when I question why God thinks I can handle this disease, and, as a former athlete, it's hard enough to watch myself get older, but watching my body be eaten up by MS is devastating. But it's my reality to embrace, and I continue to pray for the ability to see the bigger picture in this long-lasting trial. It's hard to keep from sounding ungrateful, but there are low points and real battles. Still, I am very grateful and do see new victories each day.

——————— ▣   ▣   ▣ ———————

I had been training on my own at a local gym for a few months and quietly (okay, not so quietly) doing my own routine when one of the personal trainers came over to me during a workout. Now, I'm not an easy guy to approach when I'm working out. I'm very focused on what I'm doing, and I don't say much to anyone. I keep my ear buds in and get the job done. Kendra tells me I look mean and that people probably think I'm not a nice guy. I just view it as extreme concentration. I'm there to accomplish a goal, and, if I get distracted, I will never reach it. This trainer, however, was brave enough to interrupt me as I completed a unique exercise I'd devised using the chest press machine. He introduced himself as Frank Duran and apologized for interrupting me. He was very polite and simply stated that he'd never seen anyone do what I was doing and that he wanted to know what part of the muscle was being worked.

Frank was a big guy. At first glance, he looked to be between 230 and 240 pounds, about six feet tall, and thirty years old. He was in great shape, but he was intrigued by this old man, so I explained my exercise and had him try it. He was impressed that simply by putting a bar strategically in the machine, holding his elbows a certain way, and keeping the movement in a specific line, he could work his muscles in a way he'd never done before on that device.

Frank was curious and asked me how old I was. When I said I was fifty-three, he thought I was kidding. He said he wouldn't have pegged me for anything over forty, and he told me I looked great. I didn't think

I looked quite that young, but it was nice to hear. Even if he was just kissing my butt, I was happy to get the ego boost.

After he was finished with the trial reps, I dismissed him and said I had to get through my workout; but from then on, every time I came to the gym, Frank would make it a point to say hello.

As the weeks passed by, I noticed that Frank was having his clients watch some of the exercises I was doing. He was clearly fascinated by my routines and thought they were good enough to serve as professional examples. It wasn't long before Frank came over and asked if he could train with me. Having trained on my own for so long, I was reluctant to agree, but there was also a part of me that wanted to relive the good ol' days of killing my training partner.

I explained to Frank that I had MS and that, although I would seem uncoordinated at times and have trouble grasping the bars, he could never baby me. The look on his face when I told him I was disabled with MS was priceless. His first response was, "No way do you have MS!" Followed by, "I can't believe it." Then, "How can you look this good and train as hard as you do with MS?" Poor Frank. What a can of worms he opened with all of that.

I started with my story and the MS Bodybuilding Challenge and then went into preacher mode telling him where Christ had taken me. Typically, I'm a very quiet guy—until you get me started, then I don't shut up. When I finally completed the story of David Lyons, I could sense that Frank had his own story. He told me about his past as a gang member and the troubles he'd endured. He talked about his obesity and how he had dropped a tremendous amount of weight and become a fitness trainer. We discovered that we had much in common in many different ways, and we appeared to be a natural fit.

That day, I agreed to start working out with Frank under the following conditions: no talking except to push each other; I ran the show; no missing workouts; and no crying when I killed him. Frank agreed, and the next week we began our mission to get bigger together.

————————————— ▣   ▣   ▣ —————————————

Within the first few days, I found out that Frank was a strong guy with an incredible drive to succeed. We immediately fell into a groove, and, while I pushed him to his limit, he pushed me to mine. Week after week the weights increased, along with our training intensity. On several occasions, the training would be so brutal that, while I shrugged bar-bending weights, my balance would be a noticeable problem and my left leg would shake uncontrollably. In order to complete the sets, I had to adjust and shift my body to offset the physical obstacles, but I didn't let them stop me.

Training with someone again gave me a feeling that no words could describe, especially training with someone like Frank, who took my abuse and asked for more. I come from the old school of training in which you don't stop until you can't move your muscle or even hold the weights any more. It was a training philosophy that many of the bodybuilders in my era had adopted, and, for some reason, training with Frank brought back my memories from the eighties again.

Back in those days, when I'd trained at Mr. America's Gym, owner and Mr. America Steve Michalik was known for his insane workouts, dubbed "Intensity or Insanity," which he conducted with his protégé John DeFendis, an eventual Mr. USA, who was also famous for his level of training. In my day, I followed their system as close as humanly possible, and it took me from a guy who was 150 pounds soaking wet to a 230-pound bodybuilder with very little body fat. There were days back then when I trained with such intensity that my breakfast came back up; and once in a while, training with Frank got pretty close.

I thought about when I'd first started training with Darren after the MS diagnosis and how I had just been grateful to be in the gym. Now, with a few years under my belt, I'd returned to training with intensity. I had passed the level of just wanting to reach a goal and beat MS. In my mind, I'd taken that DeLorean back in time. True, I was a different man, but I was one with old strength regained.

Not a day goes by when I don't reach back into my memory vault—even if it's only for a few seconds—and remember the days when I looked up to Arnold, Ed Corney, and other pros, or stood in the gym with DeFendis and Torchia. I don't live in the past, but I love where I've been and enjoy embracing the memories.

Even with my newfound strength, there was no way that at my age and with MS I could train with the same number of sets and reps or the ridiculous amount of weight that I once had, but I could still train to failure. Frank and I went down that path for months with great payoff. He and I both gained size and strength and achieved lower body fat. Through our banter about who was bigger and stronger and who trained harder, we developed a mutual respect that could only be found in the gym.

Many times even today Kendra tells me, "Stop picking on Frank. He's a nice guy." But in that world, that's how fondness is expressed and respect is earned. Her advice is rooted in being kind to others, and I believe I'm doing that—just in a unique language.

Frank is a tough guy with a huge heart. He knows my goals and supports them, and he would like nothing more than to see me competing on a bodybuilding stage again. But he also encourages me in the meantime by reminding me that there are very few people who can train this hard while battling MS. It's such a blessing to have Frank remind me of the truth, because MS is still, and probably always will be, hard for me to face. It's tough to look at myself as having a crippling disease, but I refuse to let MS define me. Instead, I let it motivate me. I try to view it as something that is there outside of me trying to defeat me. It is my Goliath.

———————— ◈ ◈ ◈ ————————

Today, the day has gone by with my left leg barely lifting off the ground as I walk and with pain encumbering my body. Standing without falling to the side has taken concentration. On days like this, I come to terms with my mortality and understand the path I have chosen.

It's not the contest that makes me a winner; it's the battle along the way. My goal is to compete in a bodybuilding contest at least once more in my lifetime, be it God's will. I can honestly say that standing on a stage wearing those tiny posing trunks, oiling myself up, and flexing next to a bunch of other guys in front of a thousand spectators doesn't excite me. The excitement comes from the weights I lift and the gains I make—from the training itself and in being able to work out side by side with twenty- and thirty-year-old men and see their amazement when a man over fifty with MS shows them up. It's a pleasure to see my muscles get so pumped that the veins look like they'll explode under my skin. If you are or ever have been a bodybuilder, you can appreciate what I'm saying. And if you're disabled and are achieving a dream despite your limitations, you know what I mean.

Because the truth is that most people can't. Without the gym, I personally wouldn't be able to beat MS. Without training, my purpose would be diminished. Without the challenge, I wouldn't be David overcoming Goliath. This is where I fight my battle. This is where I stare down my giant. This is where the power of God in me comes to life and together we change the world.

THE JOURNEY NEVER ENDS

Without a dream, you die. And I'm not dying anytime soon.

The late Dr. Jerry Falwell once said, "You do not determine a man's greatness by his talent or wealth as the world does, but rather by what it takes to discourage him." That quote has stayed with me, and today I am happy to say that I rarely get discouraged anymore. I'm more focused on giving Christ the praise than ever before. I have come to believe the truth of 2 Corinthians 12:9, which says that God's power is made perfect in our weakness. And like the Apostle Paul, I can boast all the more gladly about my weaknesses so that Christ's power can rest on me.

I'll never again be the physical beast I was long ago, but that's more than just the MS; that's a basic fact of age and time. When I compete in my next contest, I want to be realistic in my quest. I want to train toward a goal but really focus on the victory of the workouts themselves.

As long as I can get to the gym, push past the MS, and train like a champion, I will win the battle.

⸻ ▦ ✠ ▦ ⸻

How often do we worry about being weak? When the struggles of life start to weigh us down, our stomachs churn, our knees quiver, our hands shake, and we feel like we don't have the strength to go on. It's not just the feeling of physical weakness that makes us tremble; many times it's the feeling that we are alone in the battle. But that's never the case. Even if no one else understands what we're going through or even if no one else is enduring the challenge with us, we are never isolated or cut off from the Lord. He remains with us through every struggle, every temptation, every tragedy, every failure, every victory.

Scripture is filled with examples of His faithfulness to His followers, and the promises that remain true for us today. While it's easier to try to draw strength from those around us and to become discouraged if no one is there, God remains faithful and strong—constant. Even if we can't see Him in the flesh, we need never doubt that He is there.

For a long time I really struggled with that. After my divorce, I felt isolated and alone. But through that time I learned to rely on Christ in ways I hadn't before. And, after that brief season was over, He blessed me with Kendra, my biggest supporter—the one who always stands strong with me. She is a tremendous blessing, and I love her more today than ever. But not even her undying love and support can compare to that of the Lord, nor should it. Kendra is only human, and she isn't capable of supplying all of my needs, just like I'm not able to supply all of hers.

Our primary source of love, strength, and affirmation should be the Lord. We should never put all of our stock in another human being who is limited in his or her capability, just like we are. Instead, in moments of tremendous fear and weakness, we should turn to Christ first, and then to others, considering their support to be extra blessings from Him. By drawing from Christ, we will find that our fears need never overcome us and that we can rejoice even in trials, letting Him know that our faith in Him is stronger than the circumstance.

If I've learned one thing through my experience with MS and the MS Bodybuilding Challenge, it's that even when it seems like the world is against you—like your friends have abandoned you and life is far from what you'd planned—you can still praise the Lord. If you rely on the Him during these hard times, He will be your strength and your rock, and He will make you strong. No circumstance in life or attack from the enemy can diminish the strength we have in Jesus. We can always stand up in our weakness and proclaim our strength in the Lord who sustains us. The key is to focus on Christ and not depend on our flesh for strength. Even at our strongest, we can't stand as strong in our own power as we can in the strength of God (1 Cor. 1:25). His is a supernatural strength that allows us to have hope and peace beyond comprehension, even in our darkest moments.

In my battle against MS, I still struggle to keep walking. I still strain to grasp objects with fingers that lack feeling, and I still labor to keep pushing when my body's fatigue seems insurmountable. My pain is daily, and my symptoms are ever present, but I know that my weakness is strength to the Lord. I praise Him daily for the things I am still able to do. I thank Him for a wife who had the compassion to marry a man with an incurable disease and for my true friends. And above all, I thank Jesus for His power and love; and, somehow, my knees no longer tremble and my heart is filled with hope.

It's a priority for me to see my life as a purposeful journey with the Lord. In some ways, MS has hardened me, and Kendra tells me I need to be more empathetic to others who are struggling. She's right, of course; I just find it challenging. I work so hard to push past my disability every moment of every day, and I seldom complain; and in a way I expect the same from others. I have zero tolerance for whining.

I look at the strength and courage of my father-in-law, J. D. Sarver, who lost his leg in the Korean war when he was in his twenties. This man, who is now in his eighties, plays golf and tennis for hours at a time. He has lived with his physical disability for most of his life; and, in the face of adversity, he still earned a living by becoming a high school coach. He had three children and was active in his church, and, as Kendra tells me, he never looked at himself as disabled or complained about his limitation. To this day his faith in Christ remains rock solid, and he leads by example.

And, of course, there is my father, who survived the torture of the Holocaust as a young man, came to the United States not knowing the language, and built a successful life for his family. Now almost ninety, he moves like a man in his forties and tells his story to the world.

Then there is Kendra, who, after suffering through a devastating marriage and divorce, now handles a husband with MS, supporting my overbearing determination to get to the gym and figuring out how to feed someone who never stops eating. It's hard on her, but she stands by me and encourages me. She is the most amazing woman I've ever known.

What makes these people different? What separates them from the ones who give up, complain about their circumstances, and have no desire to overcome their tribulations? I believe it is God's power inside them, which is something we all can have if we are willing to surrender to Christ as our Lord and embrace all that He has to offer. Through a relationship with Jesus, we can all learn to fight the fight as we stare down our adversaries.

Some will choose to embrace this, and others will choose to ignore it. Some will hear God's call and never answer. Some will spend their entire lives with downcast hearts and souls after enduring adverse life situations; all the while Christ stands at the door and knocks, waiting to be allowed in and to offer the love and strength and hope we all crave.

Not every situation is like mine, and I have both empathy and sympathy for those who cannot help themselves. My heart goes out to both children and adults who suffer at the hands of others, and it breaks my heart to watch diseases and disabilities cripple the lives of many. Seeing this type of anguish is crushing to me. But, because of what Christ has offered me in the form of strength and physical power, I will continue to serve as an example and hopefully inspire people to embrace and maximize life however it comes. While my fight may be different from that of others, it is universal in many ways. The basic principles of courage, strength, and faith are fundamental to us all. Regardless of the specific challenge, I'm standing on a battlefield just like you, and I'm using the Holy Truth as my weapon.

In Ephesians 6, we read about the armor of God:

> Therefore put on the full armor of God, so that when the day of evil comes, you may be able to stand your ground, and after you have done everything, to stand. Stand firm then, with the belt of truth buckled around your waist, with the breastplate of righteousness in place, and with your feet fitted with the readiness that comes from the gospel of peace. In addition to all this, take up the shield of faith, with which you can extinguish all the flaming arrows of the evil one. Take the helmet of salvation and the sword of the Spirit, which is the word of God. (vv. 13–17)

As I train for my next competition, I've armed myself with the Lord's armor for this battle against my Goliath, and my faith is stronger than ever. I can see a clearer picture of my role in His plan, and I am pursuing it with passion.

With the guidance of Christ and the help of Kendra and my team, I have realized that what started out as an odds-defying campaign called the MS Bodybuilding Challenge has never been about me, nor is the MS Fitness Challenge. It's about bringing glory to God and sharing His Truth. It's about helping others find faith and hope. That's why He gave me this trial.

So I admit it. I'm a stubborn man who needs an occasional smack in the face. God sure knows how to get our attention, doesn't He? He leads us to paths that take us to mountains that take us to steep climbs that take us to summits. All the while, He leads, guides, directs, strengthens, and even carries us to the top. He watches us, pushes us, and delivers us to exactly where we were designed to go—if we let Him.

I want that. I want God's power to be alive inside me. I couldn't stand a life without it, and I am so thankful that He called me to fight this good fight. And I know you want it too. Deep down, you want to be alive in Christ and able to live the abundant life that can only be found in Him. Your challenge may be different from mine. You may be facing a physical disease, emotional tragedy, or extreme life situation. You may even just be overwhelmed by the day-to-day. But if there's anything I've learned, it's that there is no giant too big for us when we have God to supply the stones.

I'm His David, and the MS Bodybuilding Challenge is the weapon He's given me. I stand before Goliath, taking aim, ready to fire for the glory of God. And it is my prayer that you would embrace your own battlefield and stand before your Goliath to do the same.

STAND BY YOUR MAN

After my first phone call with Dave, I hung up the phone and literally wrote in my diary that I thought I'd just met my future husband. I'm not usually a person who just jumps into a relationship, so this was shocking to me. But after talking with Dave, I saw in him the spirit of a warrior and a fighter. Something was very different and special about him—something I really admired and wanted in my future spouse. Most importantly, though, I saw his deep faith in the Lord and his gentle, teddy-bear side that most people don't see. He likes to be the tough-guy type, but I saw through to the huge heart underneath, and I fell in love immediately.

It's funny that a California chill person would marry a New York tough guy. Until I met Dave, I'd really never known a New Yorker. We sure had some adjusting to do, and we're still working on it today. When he gets in his protective, New-York-tough-guy mode, I get in his face and say, "Calm down, dude." He's had to get used to the "dude" talk. He smiles at that because he's never had a blonde girl half his size stand up to him. I think I took him by surprise at first, but now he just grins whenever I have to calm him down. And, honestly, I think I might have a little New York in me, too, because I sure can be feisty at times. This is why we believe God was in the midst of our meeting. I would never have gone for the biker, muscular tough guy outside of His prompting. Truly, God knows our needs better than we do.

In our emails, Dave had told me of his condition. When we first talked over the phone, he told me that MS didn't control his life and that it was no big deal. Well, of course we were in the rose-colored-glasses stage of getting to know each other, so MS was put on the backburner.

As we communicated, I fell in love with Dave's strong, driven spirit and positive outlook on life. I loved his work ethic. He reminded me of my dad, who had served in the Korean War and lost his leg after being shot in combat. I never ever saw my dad as a disabled person. He was the head football coach at a large high school in Southern California and stayed active by playing tennis. When I was younger, he would try to race me, running with his peg leg. He never complained about his situation or felt sorry for himself, and I always respected him for that, seeing it as mental and physical strength. So, when I met Dave, I saw that same type of man.

The severity of Dave's situation didn't hit me until a few years later, after we were married. That's when I saw the magnitude of how a chronic disease could impact a marriage. I was talking to someone I'd just met, and that person looked me straight in the eye and asked very slowly, "You married Dave even knowing he had MS?" At first I was puzzled, but then it hit me. Wow. Making that choice had been a big undertaking.

Some people say doing something like that takes a special person, but, to tell you the truth, I knew what I was getting into to a degree. As a career home health nurse, I had seen the effects of MS up close; I just loved Dave too much for it to scare me away. I married him knowing that his health could decline significantly someday, and, to this point, the benefits have far outweighed the risks. Not only am I married to the most wonderful man, who blesses me every day, but I'm also being stretched to become a better person myself. God tells us that we become stronger through trials because we learn to trust Him more fully. Through enduring this battle with Dave, I have seen that to be true.

When asked to write a section for this book, I really didn't know which direction to go. My heart, however, gravitated toward encouraging those who care for people with chronic diseases, because it is such an undertaking. As a nurse, I see all of the parties involved, from the caretakers to the loved ones to the person with the disease, and I see the toll it takes on each one of them. A chronic disease affects everyone from business partners to spouses, and they tend to hold in their own emotions in order to protect the ill person and not cause any more stress. But this will be detrimental in the long run, as they will eventually become empty and burned out. They need to be able to express their feelings in a healthy manner so that they can remain connected to the person with the disease and in touch with who they are inside.

Caretakers, especially, need to take time for themselves and not feel guilty about it. Many people in this role find it difficult to step away, but by taking care of themselves they can take better care of another. For instance, if I want to do something like rock climbing, which Dave can't do because of his MS, it's still okay for me to do it if that's what I need to do to fill my cup and stay true to my own desires and in touch with myself as a person.

Many times I have talked with family members of people who have chronic diseases while we're standing out in their driveways and out of earshot from the affected person. They are just yearning to have someone to talk to about their struggles, which usually involve suppressed depression and anger. I've shed many a tear alongside these family members, and I want to do whatever I can to encourage folks like us who stand beside our loved ones in their battles, knowing that it's our fight, too.

There's so much more to being a caretaker than just helping our loved ones overcome physical challenges. Personally, I can say that I was not prepared for the emotional part of the experience. Yes, Dave fights the physical part head-on, but dealing with the emotional part is a different story. While he gets great fulfillment from going to the gym and having a hard workout, I don't. In fact, when I started going to the gym and lifting weights with him, I was grumpy because I had sore muscles all the time. At first we just couldn't relate on that level, which was difficult; but I now understand that he needs this for his emotional health and that I need to do something else for mine. And, when fighting a major disease, it's important that we both engage in activities that bring us life and joy so that we can be the best for each other. I highly encourage caretakers to keep participating in activities that they enjoy, regardless of whether they have the same interests as the one suffering with the disease. Trust me, it will make you both better in the long run.

When Dave and I got together, I understood the magnitude of the disease. As a home health nurse, I had cared for many bedridden MS patients in their homes, doing everything from changing catheters to dealing with horrible bed sores. Still, I pushed aside the emotions I'd experienced from being in these environments and moved forward to marry my strong man. I put the possible negative future effects of MS in the back of my mind and buried them, knowing that each person with MS is affected differently and that Dave's healthy physical appearance might just be right. It never occurred to me early on that living with someone with MS would be that hard. And, while Dave and I are both great fighters physically and emotionally, we all have our breaking points. Both of us have experienced several along the way and have had to rely on our faith and our vows to work through the challenge.

With the ups and downs, though, I have learned so much from Dave. He's taught me how to push forward and not let the little things get you down, that life is short and needs to be enjoyed daily to the fullest, and that trusting God and releasing every worry to Him is the only way to live. Being raised Christian, I knew these things in my head, but I have had to really live them out in being married to a man with MS who has to daily trust God for the future. Certainly, I haven't been perfected in this area, but I am learning to take one day at a time and trust Him for that day. It is not easy at all, but I am sure glad we have the Lord on our side.

Being a nurse and having a trained eye sometimes isn't such a good thing for me. I can tell right away if Dave is limping more or if his symptoms are changing, and it can bring me into the sad reality of the disease. It can send me into a kind of negative spiral of worst case scenarios in which I'll wind up seeing him in a wheelchair in my mind's eye. Dave always says that he couldn't take living in a wheelchair, and I don't want that for him. That's why noticing any declines brings me into the reality that he has a major disease.

Even if he doesn't tell me, I can see when he is in more pain than usual. In those moments, it's hard to know whether to ask, "Are you hurting, hun?" or just to be quiet so that he doesn't have to think about it. The whole thing is a learning process, and each individual with each disease is different, just like knowing how to meet their needs is a daily discovery. One day Dave may be down and want to talk about the pain and numbness, and the next day he may be encouraged and just want to push forward without discussing. Truthfully, the only way to handle this is to leave it in the hands of the Holy Spirit and ask Him to guide my every action and response. It's one of the most challenging things the Lord has ever asked me to do, but it has been one of the most rewarding, as I see so much fruit in both of our lives and in our marriage.

One thing Dave and I have had to work on, specifically, has been in the area of patience with others. Dave tends to think that, because he can deal with a disease, anyone should be able to deal with their issues, regardless of what they are. I've had to explain that not all people who have struggles deal with them like a bull in a china shop. We laugh when I tell him that I've never had as much pain in my life as I have since I met him, mostly because of working out. When I get tired and sore, I tend to complain about the pain, which he has little tolerance for. Before I met Dave, I never really worked out, so I didn't really experience much pain. I tease him that his numbness is actually a blessing in disguise because he doesn't feel the muscle pain like the rest of us do, but we both know that's not the case. The fact is that Dave's reality is pain—it is his norm. That's why it's understandable that he offers little sympathy to those who whine and complain about aches and soreness.

Throughout our marriage I've had to learn to understand Dave and his pain. That was a huge adjustment as a newlywed. I had to overlook my nurse training which told me to encourage resting, relaxing, and not pushing your body too far, as it would only damage it. I had to realize that if Dave were to give in to the pain and numbness and sit home doing nothing, he would probably decline so fast and become so depressed that he wouldn't want to live. It was important for me to learn that he deals with this disease in a way that most people wouldn't, and I had to let it go and let Dave be Dave. As discouraging as it might sound, I had to decide that I'd rather have twenty years of quality life with him than thirty years of him taking it easier and not being happy at all.

Dave works out not only to get the physical strength to continue but also for his emotional health. And, don't tell him I said this, but I've actually come to agree with him. Even if it doesn't work for others, it works for him. Regardless of whether he's damaging his body by pushing it so hard, it's worth it because he is living his life to the fullest and handling the situation in the best way he knows how. Yes, his ideas go against all my training, and we've had many discussions about this, but Dave is living Dave's life—not the life of a patient in a textbook.

One day, during our first year in marriage, I visited a patient in her home. She'd suffered with MS for more than twenty years and had some other disease processes also. She was totally bedridden—unable to do anything for herself. It was like treating someone who was paralyzed. This patient had a team of caretakers that included a full-time hired professional, her daughter, and her grandchildren. My job that day was to treat bedsores that weren't healing because of her lack of mobility.

While working on her wounds it hit me: this is MS. I started to tear up as I treated her wounds, realizing that this was what could happen as a result of the disease. I tried hard to finish my visit, but the tears kept flowing. Luckily the caregiver was in the other room, so I finished up and just barely made it out of there before I got to my car and broke down in sobs. I had pushed down my fear of the future so deep that it came boiling over without my even knowing it had been there. After that visit, I soon decided that taking on MS patients was too difficult for me, so I decided to change directions in my nursing career, going back into postpartum nursing. Dealing with new mommies and babies was much less emotional for me.

One thing I've learned is that each person dealing with a chronic disease deals with it in an individual way. As loved ones involved, we need to sit back and learn how they are dealing with the disease and accept them, meeting them where they are. We should support them in the way they need, not always in the way we think is right. Imagine if I fought Dave about working out. Okay, I've tried a little. But imagine if I kept the hard attitude of "I'm right and you're wrong" and battled him on the issue. We'd be at odds all the time.

Yes, we still have discussions about pushing so hard because I for one don't want him to tear another muscle. The pictures of the bleeding underneath his skin after he tore his pec the first time scare me. Even though I didn't know him then, I don't like the idea of that happening again, and I'm sure if I'd been around, he'd have gotten a good verbal beating from me. It's just my protective nature, and I get a little angry when someone doesn't listen to good advice. But anger is probably not the best way to deal with it. I haven't mastered it yet, but I am learning to "let go, and let God." If Dave tears a muscle, we will deal with that at that time, just like we do normal everyday trials. My favorite verse in these situations has become Philippians 4:6: "Do not be anxious about anything, but in everything, by prayer and petition, with thanksgiving, present your requests to God."

Another thing I've found funny is how God brought this fast-food-loving girl into the arms of a health nut. I tease him about how his giant protein powder containers take up more room in our kitchen then our regular food. I tell him to send me to cooking school because he eats like a bear at least six times a day, and I don't enjoy cooking at all. Eating is a chore for me, and I'm incredibly picky, but, to him, eating is fun and he loves to taste new foods. Going out to eat is basically a sport to him, and like a lot of guys his next meal is constantly on his mind. Before I married Dave, I was used to maybe eating twice a day, and now I have to think of at least four meals every twenty-four hours.

I can remember one time when we first met that made me laugh. We were out to eat, and I will never forget how fast Dave devoured his food. I wasn't even a fourth done! Probably because I was doing most of the talking. But Dave was just staring at my food like a dog as if to say, "Are you going to finish that?" He was so fixated on my leftovers that he couldn't concentrate on our conversation. It didn't take him long to realize that he was dating a small eater and that he'd be getting plenty of leftovers.

Another time, when we were first dating, I reached over and took a bite of his food without asking. Oh, my. Was that a mistake! The look he gave me was scary. It was as if he was going to scream, "What the heck are you doing, woman?!" We laugh about it now, and, yes, he has learned to give me a bite here and there, but I still keep a healthy distance from his food. I don't want to disturb the bear during feeding time. See? Dealing with an MS patient is one thing, but dealing with one who is a bodybuilder is quite another!

Being able to laugh at things like that is important for both of us. Dave and I try to enjoy life because, with MS, even being able to walk is a daily gift. Even though I'm not the one with the major disease, this helps me maintain a more positive outlook on life. I try to be thankful for each day of Dave's good health, because we know that an attack can happen at any time. But God doesn't promise us tomorrow. He only tells us not to worry about the coming days, as each one has enough trouble of its own (Matt. 6:34). And, by yielding himself to the Lord, Dave has taught me to cast negative thoughts aside and pursue each day with vigor. The man is such a model of perseverance and faith, and, if he doesn't wallow in his woes, why should I?

Still, one thing I must say to anyone supporting someone with MS or any chronic disease is that it's okay to get down sometimes. It's normal to be scared and to even get mad at the disease. We are human beings with strong emotions. When those times come, take them to the Lord. Be honest with Him about how you are feeling and ask Him to lift your spirits and to show you His Truth. Ask Him to help you trust Him and then do it.

Also, it's incredibly important to have an outlet to share your frustrations and focus on something or someone else. Stay active outside of the caretaking by taking up a job, a volunteer activity or hobby, and, no matter what, do not let fear control you. This will involve trusting God in a different battle: faith for the unknown.

Don't bottle up your emotions, because they will eventually spill out in the form of depression, anxiety, or other physical symptoms such as headaches, pain, and fatigue. Prioritize your own needs, as well, because, like they say, you can't take care of others if you don't take care of yourself. It's okay to have needs and to verbalize them.

Stay open and honest with close friends, and get professional help through a therapist or support group if you need to. Sometimes just having someone to listen to you will be all you need for a boost in your emotional health.

And finally, communicate, communicate, communicate with your partner. This will be an ongoing, daily process. Sometimes you'll want to talk, and sometimes you won't. The point is to remain connected to him or her at all cost and to not allow any walls to be built. And, at the end of the day, know that God is working in you and will continue to work in you until the day you go to be with Him. "Being confident of this, that he who began a good work in you will carry it on to completion until the day of Christ Jesus" (Phil. 1:6).

I am honored and privileged to walk this journey with Dave. It has taught me to trust the Lord for each day and to release my worries about the future. And that might be the biggest blessing of all: letting go and letting God take care of the future. I am so happy and privileged to be married to such a warrior and protector and to walk hand in hand with him into the future—whatever it may hold. Dave has taught me more than I could have imagined, and I look forward to many more lessons that God will teach me through him. I only hope that I can be as much of a rock for him as he has been for me.

May God bless you all in your own personal journeys and strengthen you with His faith, peace, and hope.

Kendra Lyons

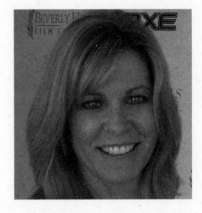

TESTIMONIALS

Darren Barnes

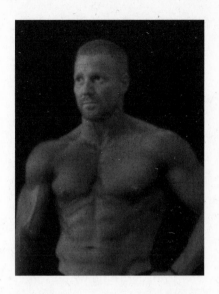

As a trainer, I have always enjoyed the challenge of helping people reach their fitness goals and improve their health. While I've had many clients in the past who each had different and unique goals, David Lyons presented a challenge like no other. When he first approached me, telling me that he wanted to begin a training program to get in competition-level shape while battling multiple sclerosis, I hesitated briefly and asked myself if I was the right person to take on this task. Was I out of my league with a challenge like this, or was this an opportunity to both help David and challenge myself?

The more David and I talked, the more I knew I wanted to take the challenge and fight this disease with him head-on. The passion David had for making his dream a reality and his determination to succeed came through in his words. He had such conviction in his voice as he described success as if it had already happened. It made me believe that if anyone could do this, it was David.

Not knowing exactly how to begin, David and I decided to train as though there was no disease and figure out how to deal with the obstacles as they presented themselves. Those obstacles turned out to be many, ranging from the neuropathy in his hands and an inability to feel the weights, to muscle tears caused by the fact that he was often unable to feel when he lifted too heavy or stretched too far. From minor injuries to major muscle tears, these injuries often forced us to make adjustments in his training. During chest workouts, David suffered many minor tears in his pectoral muscles while performing pec flies in the machine. That forced us to adjust in order to reduce his range of motion and focus less on the stretch, allowing him to perform the movement with a lighter weight while squeezing the muscle at the front of the movement for maximum contraction. But—as you have read or will read in the book—as stubborn as David was in his insistence on lifting heavy, he pushed himself to the max one day while training without me, which led to his severely torn pec that couldn't be repaired. At times like those, even when the training seemed to be going smoothly, we were given powerful reminders that the MS was there in the background threatening to derail the progress.

I remember a time during leg training when David was working with an intensity that would have made even the healthiest athlete question his ability to continue. While performing grueling sets on the leg press, I saw a glimpse of fatigue and extra effort on David's face as it seemed to take all of his remaining strength to pull himself out of the machine. The hesitation was temporary, and he immediately regained his focus as we moved to the leg extension and completed the compound set.

Through it all, David never showed signs of second-guessing his decision to compete. Instead, each setback seemed to make him more motivated to find a way to keep moving forward and finish what he started. With each workout that passed and each obstacle that was overcome, it became clear that it was only a matter of time until David's dream would become a reality.

David didn't think small. He felt that the best way to bring attention to his cause was not only to compete but to do it on the biggest stage that Florida could provide, deciding to compete at the Florida State Championship. It was a Level 5 competition in which he would share the stage with approximately two hundred other "healthy" athletes from across the state.

I would like to think that I taught David a few things about training during our time together, but the truth is that he taught me more than I could ever teach him. Each day was a lesson in character and perseverance. To see David reach his goal and step on stage was one of the most rewarding things I have ever experienced in my fitness career. When I stood backstage with him and watched as athlete after athlete approached him to tell him what an inspiration he was, I felt a sense of pride for having been a part of his success. It seemed as though many of the athletes had heard about his challenge and looked forward to meeting him. Others learned of his story only that day, by hearing the buzz that seemed to grow backstage, and felt a need to approach him and give him their support and best wishes for his ongoing struggle.

Through being part of this challenge with David, I have grown as a person as well as a trainer. I am proud to call David a friend, and I truly enjoy watching him continually make strides in his battle against multiple sclerosis.

—**DARREN BARNES**

Andrew Bishop

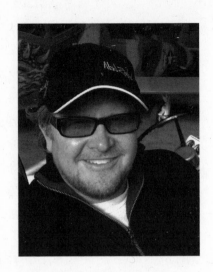

*People have been brought into my
life that forever change the way I look
at things and make life more precious to live. One day I received a
call from a friend who wanted to introduce me to someone who is in
the same business of producing television and that person was David
Lyons. Unknown to either of us at the time, that fateful day forever
changed the course of our lives as we became business partners and
best friends; together we founded Bishop-Lyons Entertainment and its
subsidiary companies.*

*The funny thing about the timing of my introduction to David is I
had just told my wife that I am ready to start another company, but
I have no desire to partner with anyone. I know this sounds self centered, but over the years many of my partnerships required me to do
most if not all of the heavy lifting and while I was prepared to go the
distance, I wasn't prepared to carry yet another person any distance,
let alone "the distance."*

*It's funny because as I write this I am sitting on the balcony of
a cruise ship while my business partner works away, so I guess my
burden of doing all the heavy lifting has past. Actually, David and
I have continually joked about how difficult it is for us to get away
from our 14-16 hour work days, so believe me it is with a heavy heart*

and a glass of champagne that I write this to a business partner who allows me to take a break. And please don't let David know this, but I will go to the ends of the earth to make sure his heavy load is much lighter, but when you partner with a former bodybuilder and fighter, they just keep adding more weight to the bar and are more happy because of it.

Arnold Schwarzenegger once said that "Strength does not come from winning. Your struggles develop your strengths. When you go through hardships and decide not to surrender, that is strength." I really believe that hardships define our character and David has a lot of character and strengths. I didn't know David prior to him being diagnosed with MS. I really knew nothing about the disease, yet my Uncle suffered from it for years when I was a child. All I knew is that this is a terrible disease with a lot of people suffering from it and yet David rarely complains, he just digs in deep and gets the work-load done. And when you are building a startup company, workload doesn't begin to define the monumental pressure and work it takes to be successful.

David has shared stories of the excruciating pain and difficulties he lives through on a daily basis and as I began to read about all the complications this terrible disease brings, the more I feel David has been blessed, even with a disease. It seems so strange to say that and yet I feel blessed to have gone through my challenges and know that I've come out a better person because of them. You see, a lesser man might not have the strength to get through the pain and make a difference for others around the world as David continues to do. "Have I not commanded you? Be strong and courageous. Do not tremble or be dismayed, for the Lord your God is with you always." Joshua 1:9

David will tell you, there are many people in the world who have it far worse than him and there are incredible stories of human spirit all around us. While others might have it "worse" than he, David is an inspiration to our team and is a man who was built to fight. He is a physically strong and courageous, but he will tell you that his spirit to fight this awful disease and make a difference is only by the grace of God.

While I've found myself in hospital beds from all sorts of injuries and ailments over the years, I've always felt blessed to get through those experiences and be relatively healthy. David on the other hand has a daily battle. One of my nastiest accidents put me in a hospital bed for six months in my living room and I found myself plea bargaining with God. 'God, if you get me through all this, I will follow you and never stray.' Well, I have strayed and even walked away from Jesus but working with David and the countless discussions we've had have made me appreciate every moment we have on this planet and brought me back to God's word in the process. We even share a number one rule for our company which is if a project falls into the "life's too short category," we don't proceed as we only want to spend our time working with people we enjoy.

Sometimes I forget that David is going through the fight of his life and that just getting out of bed in the morning is a huge task. It's very easy to forget when not only does he get up, he gets up, out the door, into the gym, and works out like a man half his age. From there, he gets into the office, takes 100+ phone calls in a day and still has time to thank the people around him. Our entire team is inspired by his daily journey and commitment to making our company a success and we often joke about him being in his twenties because he's keeping up with our twenty-something staff.

David and I are fortunate to share many of life's challenges together and I'm sure our wives would say we are somewhat married to each other as well. I guess that's how great business partnerships are nurtured to grow big, but while we've accomplished many great things in such a short time, we have only really just begun. Most importantly, through it all, I know that David has my back and I have his and God has ours. David is truly fighting his Goliath, but as Sir Isaac Newton once said, "If I have seen further it is by standing on the shoulders of giants." David is my giant and I can clearly see further because he is in my life and the future looks brighter for us all.

—**ANDREW BISHOP**, CEO/Executive Producer, Bishop-Lyons Entertainment

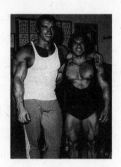

Ed Corney

As a champion professional bodybuilder who has trained for more than forty years, I know what kind of drive, determination, and intensity it takes to train and compete in the sport. It amazes me that David Lyons—diagnosed with multiple sclerosis and above the age of fifty—is able to push himself through his vigorous and exhausting regime, which would be difficult even for a young, healthy man.

I am excited to be part of the MS Bodybuilding Challenge team and look forward to seeing David continue to train and compete.

David, here are your choices: TRAIN HARDER . . . OR . . . TRAIN HARDER.

Why not? 'Cause you can!

—ED CORNEY, pro bodybuilding legend and IFBB Hall of Famer

Stan Dennis

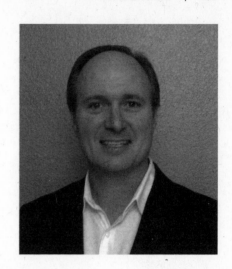

Dave and I first met years ago on the coast of Alabama when he began attending the church where I served as associate pastor. Since then, I have met very few men as driven as Dave. This has led him to succeed in many areas, including business. His entrepreneurial passion has brought him great success both in creating and working with a number of top-level companies. With that passion and with his strong desire to share the good news of the Gospel he has become a winning combination of blessing and outreach.

Currently, I serve as the National Director for FivestarMan, in which I travel across the country and come alongside pastors to help them resurrect authentic manhood in their churches. We accomplish this by focusing on five passions that already exist within every man, two of which are an adventurous spirit and an entrepreneurial drive. These two character traits have been paramount in Dave's life, and I have seen them rise to the surface in his fight against MS.

Dave's response to the doctor after hearing his diagnosis clearly illustrated his adventurous spirit. He would walk out of the hospital, never be in a wheelchair, and he would beat the disease. As far as entrepreneurship, Dave has used his business and leadership skills to go public with his fight by completing the MS Bodybuilding

Challenge and starting the MS Fitness Challenge. It's authentic man-hood in action. Now, Dave's transparency in his personal battle will serve to connect, inspire, and encourage others in whatever struggles they face.

—**STAN DENNIS**, National Director of FivestarMan.com

Frank Duran

*My story is nowhere near that
of David Lyons, but I do know
what it means to struggle. When
I started working out, I was battling significant weight issues, and my
health was at risk. Through bodybuilding, I have recaptured my life
and am now a certified personal trainer. But that is nothing compared
to what Dave must go through in his battle with MS. My weight was
controllable, and I was only fighting myself; not the case with MS. It's
an incurable disease that can't be dropped or alleviated by physical
effort and discipline. It sets your body at work against itself, so you're
up against far more than your own willpower.*

*Dave and I have been training partners for a while now, training
together four to five days per week. I've trained with many people, but
Dave definitely stands alone. Despite having MS, he gives one hundred percent. He is the most intense training partner I've ever had.
He doesn't talk much—focusing on his workouts and on spotting me
on my sets. His knowledge and training experience have definitely
helped me take my training to the next level.*

*Bodybuilding is a lifestyle, and it involves understanding your
body. It is important to train correctly, and Dave knows how to push
himself and me with proper form and intensity. One thing Dave has*

helped me to realize is how important it is to feel a muscle as it is working. Everybody says they want to feel the muscle while training, but as a trainer I rarely see them doing it. You have to think about every set, every rep, and every contraction from the first rep to the tenth. I'm still not sure how Dave does it, considering the numbness he experiences with MS, but he focuses on every movement and every rep and makes me do the same.

Our workouts don't last long—just under an hour—but when I'm done, my body and mind are totally fried. They say eighty percent of your training results come from diet, but what about the mind? I will tell you that it's a lot more than twenty percent. With such focus and determination, Dave and I push to limits I never would have imagined. And all of this is training with a guy who is twenty years older than I and has MS!

One thing I do know and will never forget is that Dave knows what he is talking about, and he didn't pick it up by reading muscle and fitness magazines. He learned from one of the best tools on the planet: experience. That's right. Dave gets his hands dirty and gets the job done in the gym. I don't look at Dave as a man fighting MS; I look at Dave as the best training partner I could ever have.

—**FRANK DURAN,** Certified Fitness Trainer

John Hansen

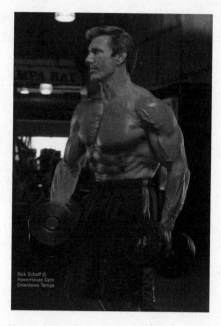

Rick Schaff ©
PowerHouse Gym
Downtown Tampa

It's so inspiring to see someone like Dave Lyons competing in a bodybuilding competition despite having to fight multiple sclerosis. Competing in a bodybuilding com-petition requires battling against weights and being disciplined enough to follow a restrictive diet. Not only does Dave train hard in those areas, he also does so while waging war against MS every day. He took it upon himself to engage in the challenge of pushing his body to the limits by competing in a contest that awards the person with the most developed body. I congratulate Dave on his amazing accomplishment, and I thank him for being an inspiration to the rest of us who have wit-nessed his incredible willpower and determination.

—**JOHN HANSEN**, Natural Mr. Olympia, three-time Natural Mr. Universe, author of *Natural Bodybuilding*

Eric Maroscher

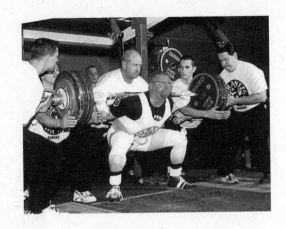

David,

Let me begin by saying that your video blew me away, and it did so for several reasons.

First, I have always said that there are two pains in life: the pain of discipline and the pain of regret. A few years ago I wrote an article for Monster Muscle *magazine called "The Choice of Two Pains." Your video gives a clear illustration of a man who chose the pain of discipline instead of sitting idly by and letting the tide choose the path. You made your own destiny and created your own opportunities. That, my friend, is why there are sheep and shepherds, followers and leaders. I love that you are making your future yours. Coincidentally, my phraseology in the closing of my letters for years has been "Ever Onward." You are clearly living your life by that mantra, and that is beyond impressive.*

—ERIC MAROSCHER, two-time WPC World Powerlifting Champion

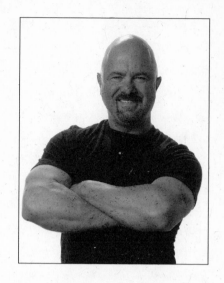

John Rowley

In this age of compromise, entitle-
ment, hypocrisy, and, for a lack of
a better word, whiners, one man
stands head and shoulders above the crowd. His name is David Lyons.

> *He is my friend, brother in Christ, confidant, and counselor.*
> *He is a loving husband to his wonderful wife, Kendra.*
> *He runs a company that is second to none, Bishop-Lyons*
>   *Entertainment.*
> *He is tireless in spreading the Gospel to all who will listen.*
> *He is in the gym daily taking care of the temple the Lord*
>   *entrusted to him.*

> *Oh, and he has multiple sclerosis.*
> *When you know David, MS becomes almost an afterthought,*
> *as the only time he talks about it is when he is helping and serving*
> *others. The MS Bodybuilding Challenge and Fitness Challenge were*
> *created so that he could bring exposure to this disease and serve*
> *those who have it. David is on a mission, and nothing will stop him.*
> *God has set him on fire for His work here on earth, and David is run-*
> *ning after it full-steam ahead.*

198 | **DAVID'S GOLIATH**

If you haven't realized it by now, this is a modern-day David vs. Goliath story. This time it is David Lyons vs. multiple sclerosis. Instead of a slingshot, the weapon of choice is iron—and lots of it.

Instead of settling for a wheelchair, David chose the gym. In fact he refuses to get into a wheelchair even on his worst days. Yes, he has up and down days, but he doesn't focus on that. He stays focused on God and the path on which He placed him. David knows that if God gave him a job to do, He will provide all he needs to achieve it.

The lesions on David's spinal cord make it difficult for him to coordinate movements and affect his balance, and the ones on his brain cause cognitive problems that damage his concentration. The lesion on his optic nerve causes him occasional vision impairment and blackness, and he lives in a constant state of fatigue.

David recently told me that he doesn't want to know about any more lesions as they multiply. "What difference does it make? The doctors want me in a wheelchair, yet God allows me to walk. I will focus on what God says, not what the doctors say about me." The fact is that David accomplishes more with MS than most people who don't struggle with anything.

Bold, brash, outspoken, and sometimes outrageous, David Lyons is a bright light in a dark world. His never-surrender attitude is needed in our world today. As you read this book, be encouraged by David's life, his example, his willpower, and his faith. Be encouraged to take action in your own life. The time is now! The person is you! So go do something!

Like David, use life's obstacles as fuel to light you on fire for the work the Lord has prepared for you.

—**JOHN ROWLEY**, ISSA Director of Wellness, author of *Power of Positive Fitness*

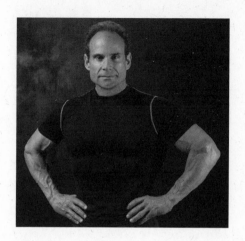

Michael
Torchia

I met David more than thirty-five years ago when I was working out with Lou Ferrigno at R&J Health Club in Brooklyn, New York, filming for the infamous 1977 movie Pumping Iron, *which featured Lou and Arnold Schwarzenegger. David was a very powerful young man who was training like a dynamo and radiating with self-confidence. When our paths crossed years later, I could see that he still possessed the same powerful physique, attitude, and energy. The only difference was that he now had MS and was battling this crippling disease.*

I truly admire David's mission to inspire other MS patients around the world to become more physically fit and active, and I am committed to helping him every step of the way. I fully support the MS Bodybuilding Challenge and his newly formed MS Fitness Challenge, and I recently incorporated David's powerful and meaningful movement with the Operation Fitness campaign. I know that together we can make a change, and, with our passion and commitment, we can make that happen.

—**MICHAEL TORCHIA**, former bodybuilding champion,
founder of Operation Fitness

"Big" Luke Wood

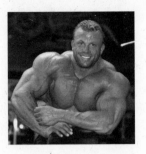

David, you are my hero and a hero to thousands of others. You are right . . . you're not in my league. You're in a league of your own—a much higher league than I will ever achieve. Not even Mr. Olympia is in your league. You are a true warrior, and may God bless you in this incredible fight. You already showed me that you can move mountains, and I know we will get those abs! You can overcome anything! Me and you and God, brother.

—**"BIG" LUKE WOOD,** six-time Mr. Australia

Author's Note:

Big Luke passed away on August 31, 2011, at the young age of thirty-five, after suffering complications from a kidney transplant. He was a three hundred-pound champion who went on to win the Mr. Australia bodybuilding contest six times after becoming the youngest bodybuilder in the world to hold a pro card. Big Luke was also a huge supporter of the MS Bodybuilding Challenge. Not only was he a bodybuilding legend, he was also a good friend and trusted source of wisdom and advice. I will miss his long emails of encouragement and his great sense of humor. Truly, his heart was as big as his muscles.

The next part of my journey will be dedicated to Luke's memory, as I am sure he will be looking down from heaven with his big smile cheering me on the whole way.

MS BODYBUILDING CHALLENGE EMAILS

The following are just a few of the many emails I have received since starting the MS Bodybuilding Challenge. Whenever I receive an email saying I've inspired someone or I get a request for advice from a newly diagnosed MS patient, I really grasp how God is using me. These emails ground me, motivate me, and, more importantly, humble me when I see how God is empowering others through my story.

Once I finally realized that my challenge wasn't just about me, I started saying that if I could touch just one life or make an impact on one person suffering from MS, I had done what God asked of me. But the truth is that it's gone beyond that. This challenge has reached thousands, and it's overwhelming for me to see the number of people who have been encouraged and changed. I'm blessed beyond what I deserve and honored to be a servant of the Lord in this battle against MS.

5/28/2012

Hi Dave,

I watched your video, and it was very encouraging. I was diagnosed with MS in November 2003, and I guess I've been doing pretty well with it. I still work part time and raise my four kids. I got on the computer this morning looking for info on muscle building, which I desperately need. I don't know what exercises to do or what supplements to take. Do you have any suggestions on how much weight to lift or where to start?

Tanya

5/15/2012
_____

I'm twenty-eight years old, and I just had a spinal tap to find out if I have MS or not. The one thing I said was, "Please don't take the gym from me." But by seeing this video, I know that even if I have MS, I don't have to lose the gym.

I get my result back this Friday. Good luck to you and your family, and may God bless you.

5/22/2012
_____

I got my results, and I have MS. They want me to start taking shots three times a week. Do you have any pointers on living with MS and weight training? Thanks for taking the time to reach out to me.

Rick

11/10/2010
_____
Hi David,

I read your inspirational story through a Fellowship of Christian Athletes mail out. I was diagnosed with the early stages of MS a little over a year ago at the age of forty-seven. As a former athlete, the cross I am having to bear has only motivated me to live a healthier lifestyle through diet and exercise. In fact, I will be running in my first Rock'n'Roll half marathon this weekend. Quite obviously, you have extensive knowledge in the area of fitness, and I would appreciate any advice you have or any references you can share regarding where to begin with an extensive weight training program and how to get the proper nutrition to battle the lack of energy I'm encountering. Thank you in advance for the inspiration and motivation you have already given me.

Stan

5/31/2012
_____
I am fifty-two years old and was diagnosed with MS a year ago. I was a competitive bodybuilder up until the age of twenty-four and continued to train until my diagnosis. When I was first diagnosed, you were a great inspiration to me, and you still are today. I never know if I will be able to get out of bed and workout tomorrow, but I will keep pushing myself because I know I'm not alone in this fight to control my body and my life.

I found out about you through an Internet search regarding bodybuilders diagnosed with MS late in life. Thank you for being there as my first source of inspiration!

Doug

10/21/2009

I have watched your video, and I am seriously impressed by your drive and determination. You think as I do. I have MS also, but I do not take any meds because I believe they will destroy my body. I do take LDN, though, as does a friend of mine who is also a bodybuilder and only believes in the natural way. Good luck to you!

Jayne

8/19/2009

I have and will pray for you and for God's favor. Know that when you step on the stage, you have already won the contest. Maybe it won't be first place in the world's eyes, but it will in God's eyes. You have set the example for others by letting them know that you could not have done it without Him, and they will be listening to every word you say and even the words you don't say. They will be watching your expressions and your body language, and I pray that the Holy Spirit will speak through you, as you witness for Him. I can't wait to hear not only how you did in the contest but, more importantly, how you affected other people for the cause of Christ. Because, when it is all said and done on Saturday, their salvation, their relationship with Him, and their eternity will be in the balance as God uses you.

Eric

8/30/09

Thank you so much, David. I know the Lord brought us together for a reason. He has blessed me in so many ways, and I owe Him everything. He also has plans for you. You stepped on that stage and did what many healthy men and women only dream of. They keep saying "next year," and next year never comes. So, to me, you are the overall 2009 Florida State champion.

Mike

10/24/08

Dear David,

I wish you much success with your challenge. I understand your struggles, as I also have MS. I was diagnosed in 2004 after I turned forty, but I'd had problems prior to the diagnosis. I too worked out very much doing power lifting and martial arts. I've been working out since I was a teenager, so it's something I would never quit. MS, though, came along and knocked me on my butt. I woke up one day and could not feel my left arm. Soon, it became partially paralyzed. I'm left-handed, so this was a huge problem. Eventually, I worked back to the point of being able to write again. I also went back to work full time and carried on with life, but I was unable to work out like I had before; I just tried to stay fit.

Unfortunately, this year my MS has gotten worse. Walking is very hard, and my left hand only opens and closes; my fingers do not work independently. The fatigue, pain, and stiffness are all very severe. It has been very tough, and I'm trying my best to continue on. I am determined to work out again someday.

When I saw your challenge, it inspired me to not give up hope of working out again. I want to say thank you for that, and I hope you make your challenge and more.

Andrew

7/7/2012

Just wanted to let you know that you are an inspiration. I was diagnosed with optic neuritis last year, and I was devastated and depressed when I was diagnosed with MS soon after. Your story has really connected with me. Maybe it's a male thing. We need to fight for our families, but this disease makes it hard as an invisible opponent. So, like you, I took a very nutritional approach: naturopathic, diet, mineral analysis, infrared sauna, vitamin D, etc. I just wanted to say that you made me look at exercise as a very important factor, and I now train three days a week. Thank you. The more we look at the release of endorphins in MS, we see that there is a therapeutic effect. I feel better, stronger, and mentally more stable. Thank you, thank you, thank you. God bless you. Luke 1:37.

R

PHOTO JOURNAL

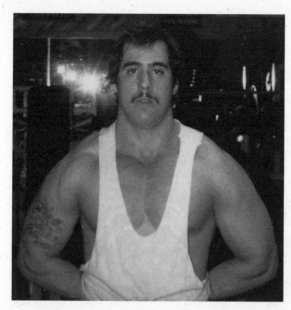

The David Lyons of the eighties. This is me at my Ultimate Bodies Fitness Center in 1983.

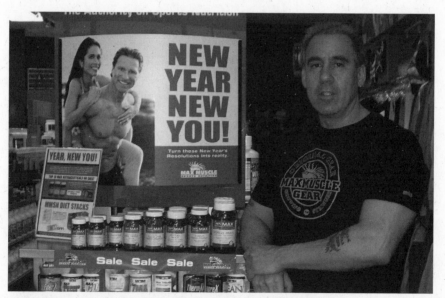

Max Muscle in Orlando was my first sponsor, and I wouldn't have been in half the shape I was without their products and support. Thanks to Ram and the team, I was fueled for the training.

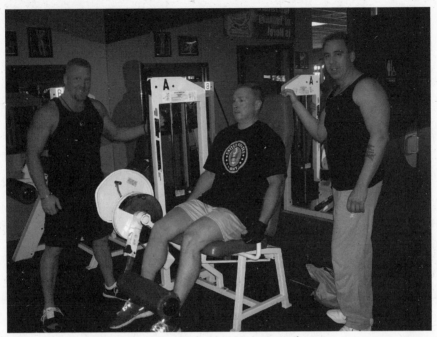

The trio that started it all: Darren, John, and me in 2008.

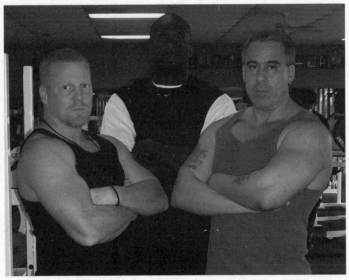

NFL veteran Greg Favors was a great encouragement to both Darren and me during our training in 2008.

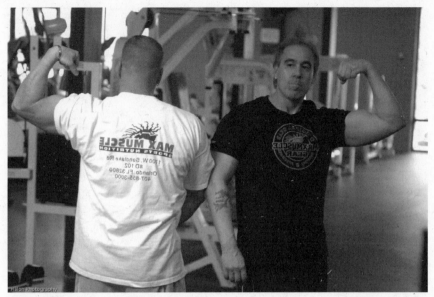

Darren and me clowning around during our first month of training in 2008. We knew how to make it lively.

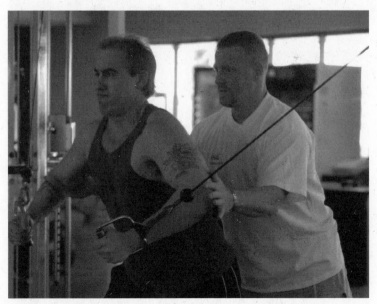

Darren's training regimen and diet plan were exactly what I needed to complete the MS Bodybuilding Challenge. His wisdom and expertise took me a long way in a short amount of time.

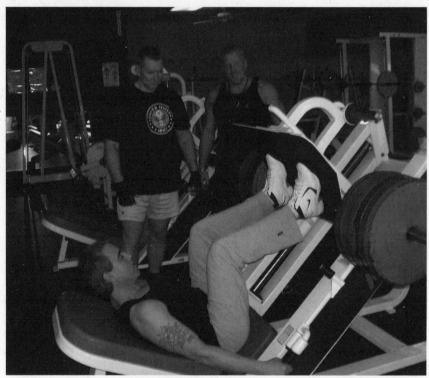

John and Darren always encouraged me to keep going. And when I look back at photos of John, I realize why I got in the car with him that day. Not only was he a State Trooper, he was also huge!

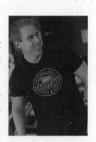

This is me during my first week of training for the MS Bodybuilding Challenge. As you can tell, I would go through many physical changes in the coming months.

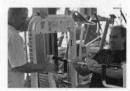

Darren was a great training partner, and I'll never be able to thank him enough for his encouragement, support, and friendship.

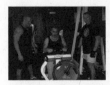

In a seated calf machine, it's normal for legs to shake under the weight, but that wasn't always the case for me. My legs shook from MS and the weight only intensified the symptom.

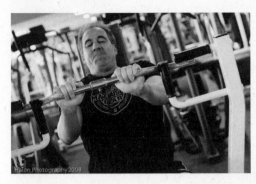

When it comes to training, I'm usually all business. I like to get in and get started, and it takes a lot to distract me when I'm in the zone.

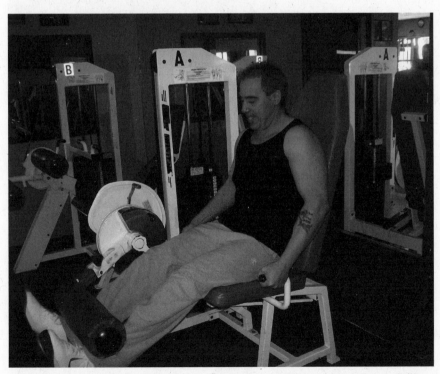

Leg extensions were never easy because of the shaking in my left leg. Still, the seated movements were easier than anything that involved standing up.

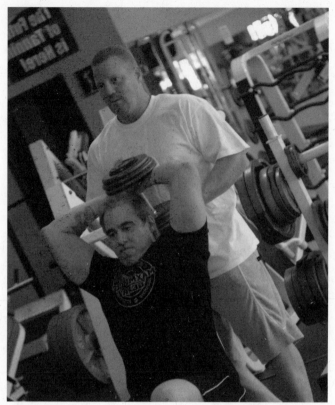

Training with "Big" Darren in 2008. He never let me
have it easy.

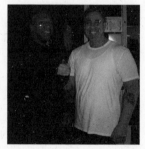

Deke Warner and me in 2008.
Without this man, I wouldn't
have been able to stand on that
stage in 2009. Thanks, Deke.

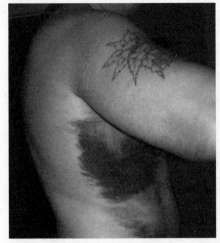

The internal bleeding of the muscle tear turned my entire right side black, blue, and red.

Because of my MS-induced numbness, I couldn't feel the pain of the torn muscle, but I sure could see the damage.

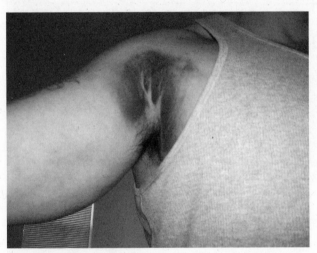

Torn pec beginning 2009: The torn pec I experienced was one of the worst my doctors had ever seen.

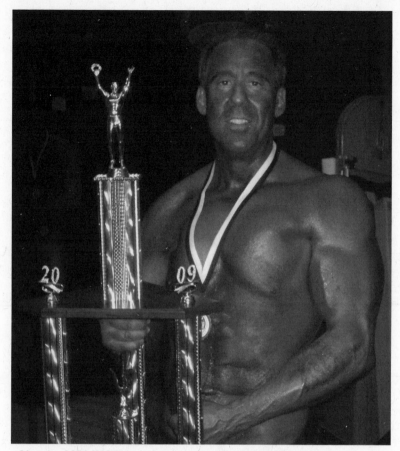

After the 2009 NPC Florida State Bodybuilding Championships, I was awarded the Most Inspirational Bodybuilder Trophy. It was a prize that meant more to me than any award I could have won for physical performance.

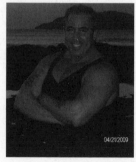

This is me in April 2009. Between this photo and the contest, I would drop a lot of mass, as you can tell.

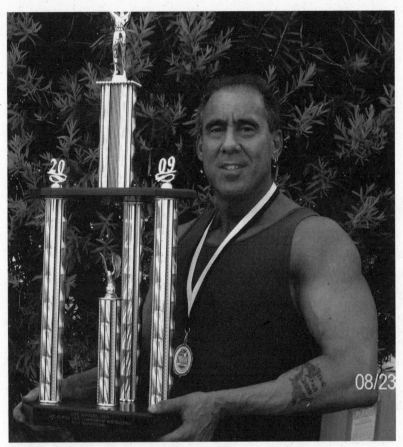

The day after the competition I was proudly sporting my medal and showing off my trophy.

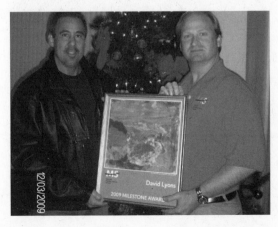

In 2009, the National MS Society presented me with their Milestone Award. The NMSS is an incredible organization, and it's been great working with them to help other MS patients move toward a healthier, more active life.

One organization that is particularly close to my heart is the Fellowship of Christian Athletes, which focuses on reaching the world for Christ through sports. In 2009, I was blessed with the opportunity to speak at an FCA Fitness camp.

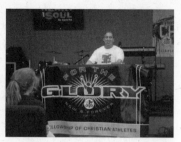

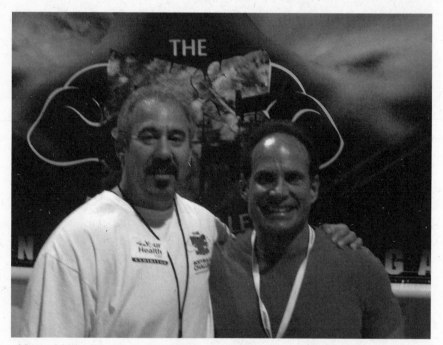

Me and Mike Torchia at the NBC Expo in 2011. Mike's been an incredible source of support, and I respect him both as a competitor and a professional.

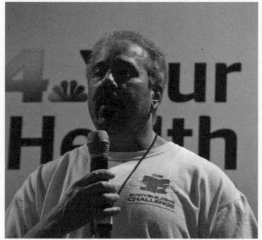

The NBC 4 Your Health Expo was a great opportunity for me to share about the MS Bodybuilding Challenge and how I've used physical training to battle the disease.

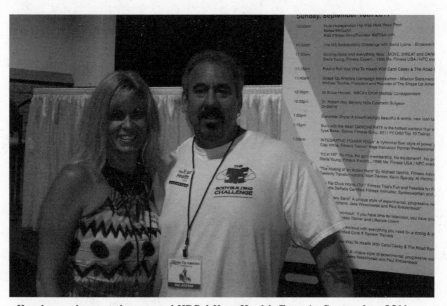

Kendra and me at the annual NBC 4 Your Health Expo in September 2011.

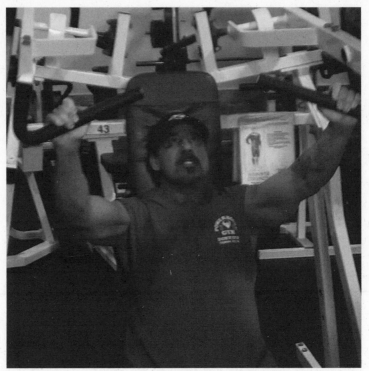

Powerhouse Gym San Jacinto CA 2011: After having to baby my chest for so long because of tearing my pec in 2008, I appreciate the workouts even more today.

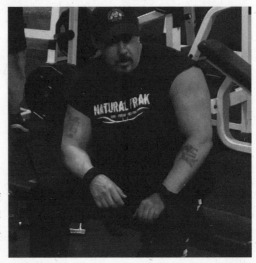

Yes, even my intense workouts require moments of rest. Here I am training at Powerhouse Gym in San Jacinto, California, in 2011.

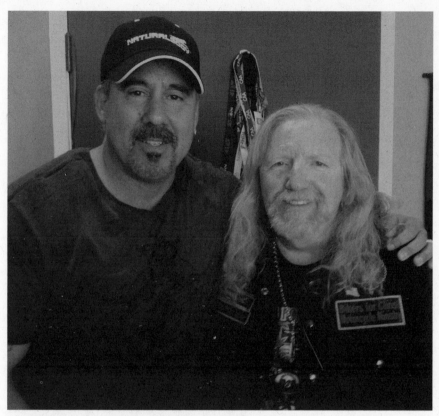

This is me with Pastor Z from Bikers for Christ. The MS Bodybuilding Challenge opened up so many doors to speak about Christ, and I loved connecting with this group.

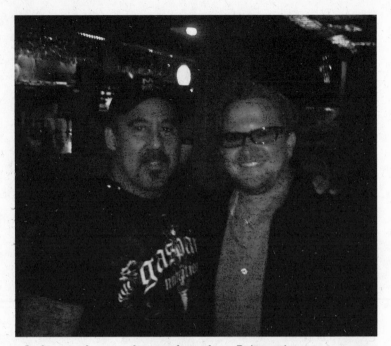

Andrew and me on the set of our show *Reinvention*.

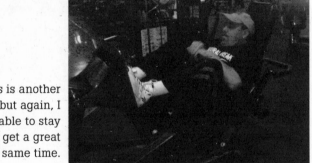

Leg press is another challenge, but again, I enjoy being able to stay seated and get a great burn at the same time.

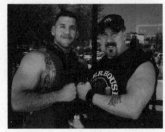

My 2012 training partner Frank Duran and me. He's a tough guy just like me, and I love it!

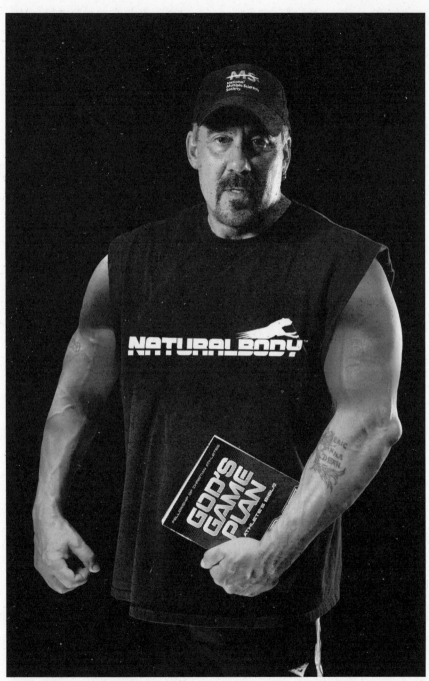

This photo represents the components of my journey: MS, training, and Christ. I'm heading into 2013 and training for the next competition.

WEB RESOURCES

THE MS BODYBUILDING CHALLENGE
themsbodybuildingchallenge.com
davidlyonsms.com

THE MS FITNESS CHALLENGE
msfitnesschallenge.com

NATURALBODY
naturalbody.tv

BISHOP-LYONS ENTERTAINMENT
bishoplyons.com

FELLOWSHIP OF CHRISTIAN ATHLETES
fca.org

NATIONAL MS SOCIETY
nationalmssociety.org

POWERHOUSE GYM
powerhousegym.com

PLATINUM NUTRITION
www.facebook.com/platinumnutritiononline

HIGH ENERGY LABS
highenergylabs.com

THE BIGGEST LOSER RESORT
biggestloserresort.com

MAX MUSCLE NUTRITION
orando.maxmuscle.com

INT'L SPORTS SCIENCES ASSOC (ISSA)
issaonline.edu

GASPARI NUTRITION
gasparinutrition.com

BIOTRUST
biotrust.com

JOHN ROWLEY
peakperformancelifestyle.com

MICHAEL TORCHIA
  operationfitness.com
JOHN HANSEN
  naturalolympia.com
ERIC MAROSCHER
  monstergaragegym.com
BRAD HOMAN, DO
  celebrationorthopaedics.com/physicians/brad-homan-do
DR. JASON KELBERMAN, DC
  drkelberman.com
MONICA CALLAN, RD, CPT
  organized-wellness.com
DEKE WARNER
  npcfloridastate.com
CLAY WALKER
  bandagainstms.org
ED CORNEY
  edcorney.net
DARREN BARNES
  dbarnes2254@yahoo.com
STAN DENNIS
  stan@fivestarman.com